FB e ChoiceCommunity.com
Website.

Pregnancy and Abortion – Your Choice

'There seem to be two images of women who have an abortion; cold-hearted . . . who have the abortion as easily as having a tooth out, another form of contraception, or victims racked by depression, guilt and regret.

'The truth lies somewhere in between. It's not an easy decision to make. It's somewhat more complex than having a tooth out.'

Anne Marie, *Girl Frenzy No. 6, quoted by Germaine Greer* in
The Whole Woman

Pregnancy and Abortion
Your Choice

Dr Mark Houghton
Dr Esther Lüthy
Professor John Wyatt

malcolm down
PUBLISHING

First published 2017 by Malcolm Down Publishing Ltd.
www.malcolmdown.co.uk

British Library Cataloguing in Publication Data
A catalogue record for this book is available from the British Library.

ISBN 978-1-910786-80-2

IMPORTANT MEDICAL NOTICE

Every care has been taken to ensure accurate information in this book. But this
book is not a substitute for personal medical advice to any reader. Any reader
wishing for medical advice should consult his or her own medical practitioner
in matters relating to their health and specifically with respect to any symptoms
that may require diagnosis or medical attention.

Before any form of medical treatment, you should always consult your personal
medical practitioner. In particular, (without limit) you should note that advances
in medical science occur rapidly and some information about procedures, drugs
and treatment in this book may soon be out of date.

Cover design by Mantra Media, Sheffield
Art direction by Sarah Grace

Printed in Malta

Dedication

To all pregnant women and their near relations

Acknowledgements

Pregnancy, abortion, adoption and parenting are complex issues bringing us face to face with health, hope and happiness but also with hatred, dilemma and darkness.

First, thanks must go to the patients who have trusted me with their hearts and lives over the last 40 years. I can't name you but I appreciate you.

No person can know and make sense of all these issues on their own. I am in debt to a small army of women and men, from the very young to the very old, some 'ordinary' people and several world-class experts in their field.

Many have shared their stories, so names have been changed to protect their identities.

Thank you one and all for your endless patience with my fountain of questions and interruptions: my family, Dr Esther Lüthy a tireless cowriter, a female pregnancy counsellor, Fiona Campbell PhD, Polly Paffard, Philippa Taylor, Janet Gillham, Hilary Jones, Esther Johnson and her lovely study, Dr G. Gardner, Dr Fiona Fairlie on fetal medicine, Professor John Wyatt, Dr P. Saunders, Dr G. McAll, Dr T. Gray, Ali Hull with Mark Finnie and their Lakes writers' weeks, Professor Joel Brind PhD, Dr P. Caroll, Brent Rooney, K. Neeley, Brigid Houghton and Benjamin Houghton, Dr R. Dixon statistics, Revd Dr B. Cooper worldviews, Dr Janet Goodall, Dr Kirsty Saunders, Sharn Johnson, Sally Thomas copy-editing, Grant Lynas illustrator – and finally those too many to name here.

Malcolm at Malcolm Down Publishing, has been a steady hand on the wheel steering this project with his great experience towards conclusion - many thanks indeed.

I think we have all striven to dig out the truth from wherever it is buried, but at the end of the day the results are my responsibility and factual corrections in this fast changing scene will be online.

Personal Note from the Author

Dear Reader

This book is written to help you make your own choice about an unintended pregnancy that you are unsure about, or check things even when sure.

While writing this book I was amazed to discover what a big subject this is. I am driven by a desire to pass on these findings for your benefit.

Every woman or couple deciding together deserve the best information. Information is essential to help you make an informed choice and to liberate your free and lawful rights.

This book is about the choices in front of you when you find yourself pregnant. It looks especially at what abortion entails and the personal and family risks to weigh up. The information is not to judge or blame it's to help you think it through.

While these issues trigger many emotions, we have tried to be objective, to leave you free to think and choose. And you don't have to read the whole book to find what you need.

Thinking over the pregnancy decision, often under pressure from time and other people, can be very difficult. So, in Part 1, an experienced female pregnancy counsellor helps you move forward to a decision. Take your time over this. It's not easy to weigh up choices when your head and your heart may be saying different things. In Part 2 you can explore your options, and more in-depth information on abortion and the results of research come in Part 3.

I hope this book helps you reach the conclusion best for your situation, now and in your life ahead.

Mark Houghton, lead author

Contents

Introduction

Sex is one of the greatest pleasures humans enjoy together. But an unplanned or unwanted pregnancy can bring a sense of shock and confusion, which may affect your ability to think clearly about what to do next.

If you find yourself in this situation, this book will help you decide what to do. It is also for friends, family and people supporting you in the deciding process.

It may be that you thought you knew immediately what you wanted for the pregnancy when you found out about it but since have become unsure. You may have opened this book to help confirm the decision you have already made or to look up a question you have.

Follow the map

We offer a reliable, proven and convenient method for making choices, along with the knowledge you will need, all in one place.

Imagine you are travelling from Manchester to London by country roads – without the latest sat-nav you would soon get lost. If you are not sure what decision to make regarding your pregnancy, the first part of this book is like a roadmap to support you. It provides tools to help you make up your mind. The second part goes on to give you more information about the options you have.

As with any medical procedure, you should find out as much as possible about the known complications (after-effects) of both birth and abortion. We talk about and compare the short-term and long-term effects of parenting, adoption and abortion. However, for the purpose of this book, giving birth (which is well covered elsewhere) and adoption are not covered in as much detail as abortion.

The third part goes into much more depth, exploring much of the research that has been done on the physical and emotional after-effects of abortion in particular, that can affect those who have had an abortion and also their partner and family.

Your inner map

Everyone has beliefs and values (even having no beliefs can be a kind of 'belief'). Beliefs about abortion can be used to pressure you either towards or away from abortion. Look out for this pressure from anyone who is giving you support or advice. It is easy to give an opinion when you are not in the driving seat.

As a writing team, our aim is to put the choice in your hands. The decision is yours and should be true to who you are. This is vitally important for your ongoing life and emotional wellbeing.

How to Use this Book

This book is intended to help you in making decisions about pregnancy, birth, abortion and adoption. But it is not a substitute for professional help. A word of caution however: professionals, friends and family may urge you to make a 'choice' you don't want. Even family doctors and school nurses may push either abortion or birth. This guide helps you step back, take control and tell them what *you* want – it's your choice, *always*.

Navigating this book

Part 1 is a counsellor's guide, taking you step-by-step to a decision, using the 'Journey to Decision' tool. Chapters 1 and 2 cover how to confirm pregnancy and how to keep calm and see what to do next. Chapters 3 to 6 map out the journey to a decision in four steps, so they are best read one after the other.

In Part 2 we explore the different options you have and give you information that you may want to consider as part of your decision-making process. In Chapter 7 we take a look at how the unborn baby develops week by week and in Chapters 8, 9 and 10 explore the implications of parenting, adoption and abortion.

In Chapter 11 we have a look at the law on abortion; Chapter 12 looks at the negative after affects that can be experienced post abortion.

Teenage pregnancy and the extra special care that needs to be taken when considering options is covered in Chapter 13; how unexpected pregnancy and your choices may affect the father is considered in Chapter 14. In Chapter 15 we investigate the antenatal tests you are offered when pregnant and the tricky questions surrounding possible disability in the fetus.

Part 3 looks at abortion in much more depth, digging deeper into the years of research that has been carried out looking at both the short-term and long-term after effects. If you are considering abortion, then it is worth checking out all the pros and cons before coming to a decision.

In the appendices at the back of the book you will find 1) a summary of the different beliefs about abortion held by some of the main religions, 2) a handy guide to where you can find help, whatever your situation, and 3) a glossary of the medical terms used in the book.

Part 1
The Journey to a Decision

Chapter 1
Am I Pregnant?

This chapter covers:

- Pregnancy tests

- Pregnancy – what happens inside you?

- Pregnancy symptoms

- Pregnancy without full intercourse

- Pregnancy with contraception

- I'm pregnant – what now?

Pregnancy Tests

First things first. It's essential to be sure whether you are really pregnant or not. Periods can be missed for other reasons than pregnancy. Emotional upsets and minor illnesses can cause a missed period. Equally, light bleeding or spotting of blood can seem like a period when in fact it is the first missed period of a pregnancy. Remember to make a note of the date of your last menstrual period (LMP) – perhaps on your phone – as this could be useful later.

A simple test on a sample of your urine will give a reliable answer as to whether you are pregnant or not. Kits are available from pharmacies. You will need:

- to wait until the day of your missed period.

- an early morning urine sample.

Standard pregnancy tests show a pregnancy by detecting the pregnancy hormone HCG in a woman's urine after she falls pregnant.

Getting a Pregnancy Test

Your local pharmacy can supply a test kit for about £1.50.

Some pharmacies will test on site.

NHS family doctors or nurses in a GP practice will do a test free of charge.

Pregnancy tests are most reliable from the first day of your missed period – that means the one expected but missed. More expensive tests can work as early as 4 or 5 days before your period is due.

How reliable are pregnancy tests?

A *positive* test (saying you are pregnant) is almost certainly correct.

A *negative* test (saying you are not pregnant) is not so reliable. If your test is negative then it is best to test again in 2 or 3 days. If you keep getting negative results but you think you could be pregnant, see your doctor.

If you get a positive test on the first day of your missed period, it's probably about 2 weeks since you conceived.

Pregnancy tests done on a sample of your blood can be positive a few days before the urine pregnancy test and can be obtained from your GP.[1]

Pregnancy – What Happens Inside You?

A woman releases an egg monthly and this is called mid-cycle ovulation (the release of the egg from the ovary). Fertilisation (falling pregnant) happens about 8 days before the woman's next expected period.[2] Implantation of this embryo in the womb usually happens 6 to 12 days after mid cycle ovulation.

A positive blood test for pregnancy can occur as early as 3 to 4 days after you see some slight implantation bleeding, and 4 or 5 days before a missed period.[3] This sort of bleeding – or 'show' – can be mistaken for a period.

Pregnancy Symptoms
There are some other clues that can indicate pregnancy. These include:

- Stomach cramps

- Urinating more often

- A strange metallic taste in the mouth

- Feeling very tired

- Feeling sick, often in the mornings but also at other times of day

- Breasts becoming larger and more sensitive

RED FLAG

Ectopic Pregnancy
If you have persistent abdominal pain in early pregnancy, please call a doctor the same day. This is to exclude the possibility of a serious condition called 'ectopic pregnancy', where the fetus is growing in the wrong part of your body. Untreated ectopic pregnancy can threaten your life.

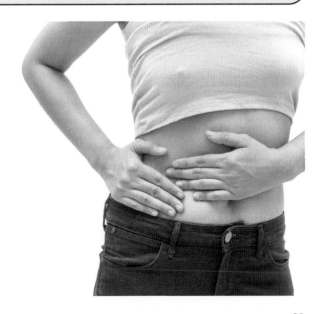

Not everyone will experience all pregnancy symptoms and it may be that you have experienced none of these but you are still pregnant.

Pregnancy Without Full Intercourse

It may be you're thinking you can't be pregnant because you didn't have full intercourse, for instance if your partner withdrew from you before climax. However, it is still possible to become pregnant through this kind of foreplay, since some sperm may have been released.

Pregnancy With Contraception

It maybe you're thinking you can't be pregnant because you were using contraception. Whilst contraception is very effective under *ideal* conditions, it does fail sometimes.

Here are just a few reasons why contraception can fail:

- The condom can break during intercourse.

- The contraceptive pill may not work effectively, especially if you are on certain medication like some antibiotics.

- The morning-after pill (MAP) can fail also.

Surely not me!

If you have had sex or intimate foreplay in the last 3 months, you could be pregnant, even if you used contraception.

I'm Pregnant – What Now?

Read the next chapter 'Pregnant – What Next?' which will get you ready for our self-help guide to making a choice.

Chapter 2
I'm Pregnant – What Next?

This chapter covers:

- My thoughts and feelings

- My body

- Tunnel vision

- Preparing for the journey ahead

My Thoughts and Feelings
Let's assume from now on that pregnancy has been confirmed. You may have a lot of questions, such as:

- Why is this happening?

- Why me?

- Why now?

Feelings of disbelief are often the first response. There may be issues around whose baby this is, who you want to tell or not tell, and what other people's responses will be.

On the other hand, you may just feel numb and unable to think or respond. Or you may be feeling relieved that you can get pregnant or happy that you are pregnant. There is a wide range of initial responses.

The key thing is to give these feelings a few days to settle while you process what has happened and think things over. It may be helpful to talk over your situation with someone you can trust. Or you may feel easier talking about it with people who are not part of your everyday life (see Finding Help on page 173).

My Body

Within hours of you becoming pregnant, your body will have begun to change. Pregnancy releases hormones all over your body that may affect your emotions. As your body adapts, you may experience ups and downs in your mood from one minute to the next. It is not uncommon to feel times of high elation and then to plummet to tearfulness and confusion. No one can tell you exactly how you are going to feel through this time, as hormonal changes affect women differently.

Mood swings

As your body changes and adapts to pregnancy you may experience dramatic changes in your general mood. Such emotions can add to the confusion you may be experiencing in your thinking. They can make it even more difficult to decide. They can add to uncertainty and to swinging from one decision to another.

Tunnel Vision

The shock of an unexpected pregnancy, like any other shock, can suddenly change your outlook on life. You may feel unable to cope. This may plunge you into a dark tunnel where the only light seems to be at the other end of the tunnel. You may expect to only surface into the brightness of everyday life once you have made up your mind.

This 'tunnel vision' can produce a strong desire to turn the clock back, but the track is going one way only, and the reality is that your life at the other side of this decision will be different to life before. Whatever decision you make, this will become part of your life experience.

'Tunnel vision' can also plunge anyone pregnant into panic as the decision-making comes nearer. You may feel separated from the inner resources you would normally use to deal with difficult life situations. You may find it hard to imagine life on the other side of the tunnel.

Getting to grips with the short chapters called 'Making Choices' will help you find your inner strengths and apply them to your problems and challenges. It will also help you to see the bigger picture. Even if you're not feeling shock or panic, you may still want to work through these four steps in Chapters 3 to 6. You can use the rest of the book to find out more information and check out facts, before you make your final decision.

Preparing for the Journey Ahead

In this adjustment phase, you may find questions swirling round your mind. See if you can tease out what they are and try writing them down.

Questions you may ask yourself

- How am I feeling?

- Am I ready to be a mum?

- What will *my* mum/dad/partner/children say?

- What options do I have?

- What do I know about these options?

- Where can I get help?

- What am I going to do?

The rest of this book is designed to help you to work through these questions and find some answers.

Chapter 3
Making Choices 1
The Journey to Decision

This chapter covers:

- Feeling the pressure

- Introducing the Journey to Decision

- Preparing to start

Feeling the Pressure

You may find making choices difficult at the best of times, but a pregnancy decision can be overwhelming. You may only just be getting your head around the shock of finding out you are pregnant and feel in no fit state to choose what to do.

If you have shared with others that you are pregnant, you may have had some very strong reactions from your partner, friends or relatives offering you their advice. Or you may have 'I'll support you whatever you decide' ringing round your ears and just wish you could turn the clock back and not have to make the choice at all.

You may already be feeling sick and weepy, with your hormones going crazy. On top of all this, there is the mounting pressure of time ticking away: every day you delay, the pregnancy is moving forward. Under such pressure, and with such conflicting feelings, how do you begin to think about what to do?

Introducing 'The Journey to Decision'

The feeling of being confused and unable to cope is a normal response to the shock of an unplanned pregnancy.

The following picture illustrates a helpful tool called 'The Journey to Decision'. Put yourself at the start of that journey rather than at the 'Roundabout of Decision' where all the pressure falls. There is a whole journey to go through before you arrive at the roundabout and must make the decision.

Hopefully, the journey will begin to make things clearer for you. Don't worry too much about how long it takes; the different stages on the journey can sometimes be completed in less than a day and sometimes weeks. The time it takes *you* to complete this journey is individual to *you*.

[see diagram on opposite page]

Preparing to Start

You will need a quiet space, and pen and paper. As you can see in the picture, there are five stages: the first 'Explore situation' helps you to look at your situation from lots of different angles (Chapter 4); the next three 'Look at options', 'Gains and losses' and 'Information' (Chapters 5) help you to look at the options in front of you. The final stage 'What next?' (Chapter 6) is about planning your next step.

You may want the support of a trained pregnancy counsellor to help you apply some of the tools to your own situation, or you may want to turn to a trusted adult friend. Since it involves some writing down, you may just want someone to do that for you whilst you talk. It is important that after you have worked through the stages of the Journey the decision you come to is your own.

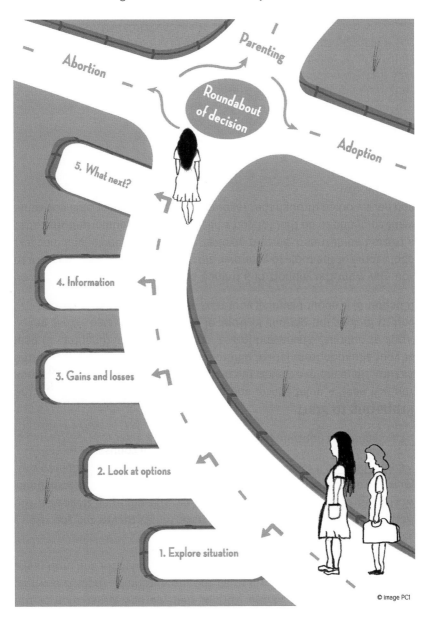

© image PC1

Chapter 4
Making Choices 2
Exploring Your Situation

This chapter covers:

- Exploring your situation

- The 4H tool:

1. What's happened?

2. What's going on in your head?

3. What's going on in your heart?

4. What are you bringing in your hands?

- Reviewing your situation

Exploring Your Situation

This chapter just covers the first step on the journey to decision: exploring your situation from lots of different angles.

Pregnancy situations can be so difficult because there are often lots of things going on at different levels that can cause conflicting thoughts and feelings. Here we try to unpack what those conflicts are about, to make things clearer for moving forward.

Claire's story

Claire is 20 years old, in her second year at university and enjoying her studies. She has been on the pill but forgot to take it a couple of times and has just found out she is pregnant. She has only known her boyfriend for six months and doesn't want to tell him. Her mum was pregnant as a teenager and had encouraged her to go on the pill, so she doesn't want to tell her either. She feels devastated that this has happened and annoyed at herself. She is thinking of having an abortion.

The 4H Tool

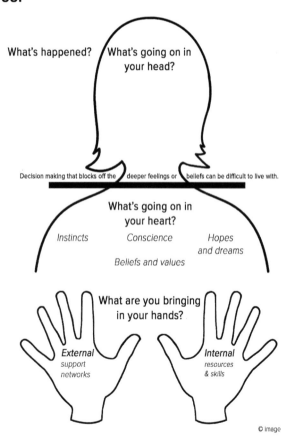

What's happened?

What's going on in your head?

Decision making that blocks off the deeper feelings or beliefs can be difficult to live with.

What's going on in your heart?

Instincts   Conscience   Hopes and dreams

Beliefs and values

What are you bringing in your hands?

External support networks

Internal resources & skills

© image

The tool contains four words beginning with 'H' that represent different parts of your situation, as shown in the diagram above.

1. Happened

2. Head

3. Heart

4. Hands

The first and the last (Happened and Hands) are more about what is going on in your outside circumstances; the middle two (Head and Heart) are exploring what is going on inside your mind and at a deeper level inside you.

> At the end of the chapter you will find a completed diagram, using Claire's situation as an example, and a blank diagram for you to fill in yourself.

1. What's happened?
'What's happened?' may seem like an odd question. You obviously know what's happened and don't need to write it down. If you are working through this with someone, it is helpful for them to know what's happened. For your part, write around the top outside space around the head (as in the completed example) all the circumstances or the things that have happened that are making this pregnancy difficult for you.

Be very specific and put down the *facts* of your situation. You may be very young, in full-time education, have a good job, not sure who the father is, have no money, no plans to have a child now, etc. You may have several circumstances that are making you anxious. List them all.

2. What's going on in your head?
Our mind interprets for us the things that are going on around us, and the head represents what we are telling ourselves about what is happening. What thoughts are constantly going through your mind about this pregnancy? Write inside the head space what you are thinking. Try to identify the thought patterns that keep being repeated inside your head

and why you're thinking what you're thinking at any one time.

You may be telling yourself, 'No one must know,' 'I'm going to lose my partner if I don't make a certain decision,' 'I couldn't manage,' 'I don't want a baby now,' 'My parents will kill me!' 'How could I be so stupid?' It may be that you're feeling sure about what you want to do.

Once you have written down your thoughts, pause to consider a few things:

- If you are feeling pressure, where is that coming from?

- Is it genuine pressure or what you are anticipating may happen?

- What would need to change to release some of that pressure?

- Are you feeling that you have a genuine choice?

Whether you feel it or not, there is a choice and it belongs to you.

3. What's going on in your heart?

The 'heart' is referring to anything that is happening inside you at any deeper level. This may include your instincts, your beliefs and values, your hopes and dreams, and motivations. The heart holds those things that are usually deep-rooted within us and helps to define who we are and how we see ourselves. It helps us to shape where we want to be in 5 or 10 years' time. Ask yourself, is there anything else going on for me at any other level regarding this pregnancy?

It may be that when you first discovered you were pregnant you were excited. You may have started to connect with this pregnancy and are already thinking and imagining the future if you were to continue. Perhaps you have always wanted a baby but the timing is difficult. You may have had strong beliefs and values about pregnancy and abortion before you became pregnant that you are now thinking of going against. Maybe none of these applies to you, but you may recognise that there are some uncomfortable thoughts or feelings surfacing as you consider a particular option. Write all these in the Heart area – anything that reflects deeply held values.

Decision-making that involves every aspect of our lives will generally lead us to decisions that we can live with. When the head and the heart agree, there is no internal conflict about the course of action. Decision-making that blocks off deeper feelings and beliefs (when those are different to what our mind is rationalising) can be difficult to live with. It is then more likely to lead to problems afterwards. The support provided to those who have had an abortion confirms this.

Ask yourself, does anything in your Heart area conflict with what is in your Head area? If so, think about the decision in terms of how you may feel if you go against your heart? How will that affect you as a person? How might that affect you in the future?

4. What are you bringing in your hands?
This is about who or what you have to support you in this situation, including your own strengths and weaknesses.

Use one of the hands to write down what your *external* support networks are, such as partner, family, friends. Put here, too, any support you are getting from organisations, such as social care or counselling. Are any of these support networks relevant to your decision? If yes, in what way?

Use the other hand to write down what *internal* resources you are bringing to the situation – or feel you *don't have*. This could be an aspect of your personality, such as being determined, independent – or maybe prone to depression, struggling with mental health. It could be a relevant skill, such as you are very good with children – or not very good with children. You might like to photocopy the 2 pictures on the following pages, so you can fill in your thoughts on the blank picture.

Reviewing Your Situation
When you have finished filling in the blank 4H tool, pause to read over it and consider what you have written:

- Has it helped you to clarify where you are at and what you are bringing to this situation?

- Look particularly at any conflicting feelings that have come up. Is there a way of resolving those feelings?

- Are you feeling any nearer to making a decision?

This is the just the first step on the journey to decision-making. Keep going until you reach the roundabout. The next three steps take a thorough look at the choices facing you.

What's happened?

20 years old.

2nd year at University - enjoying studies.

Boyfriend - student known for 6 months only.

Been on Pill but forgot to take it a couple of times.

2 weeks overdue - done test and pregnant.

Can't tell Mum, she was a pregnant teenager and wanted better for me.

Was enjoying life - now feel devastated.

What's going on in my head?

An abortion would mean I don't have to tell my boyfriend or my mum and I can carry on with my studies.

I feel stupid because it's my fault for forgetting the Pill - it's the wrong time and the wrong place to be having a baby.

I never thought it would happen to me.

What's going on in my heart?

I've done lots of crying - I had plans to have a baby but not like this.

I've not been drinking because I'm pregnant.

I've never been against abortion for others but I don't think I'd do it.

I feel I've let myself down and everybody else.

I feel guilty about not telling my boyfriend - not sure what this will mean for our future.

What are you bringing in your hands?

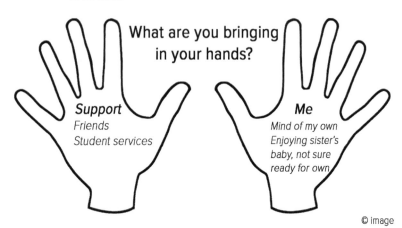

Support
Friends
Student services

Me
Mind of my own
Enjoying sister's baby, not sure ready for own

© image

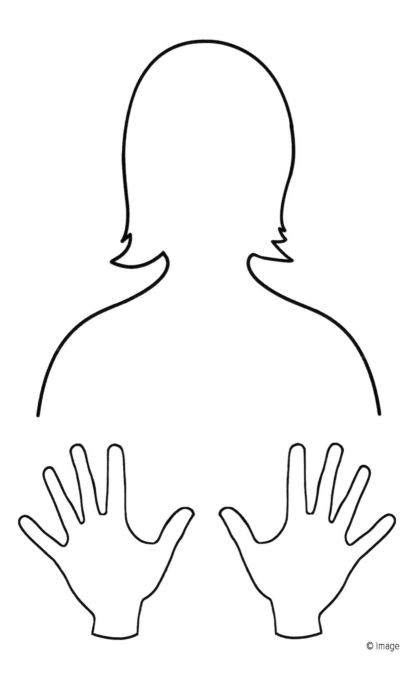

© image

Chapter 5
Making Choices 3
Looking at the Options

This chapter covers:

- Looking at options

- Weighing the gains and losses of each option

- Making an informed decision

Looking at Options

There are three possible choices when faced with an unplanned pregnancy – parenting, adoption or abortion. The Journey to Decision encourages you to consider them all and what each would mean in your situation. The order in which you consider them depends on you. If you don't want to look at one of these options, think about why not. Adoption is often the option that people find the most difficult to consider and is the last route off the roundabout for that reason.

However, for someone who feels that they cannot parent yet but doesn't agree with abortion, it may become the best option.

On a sheet of paper, make three columns with the three choices as headings, like the ones shown in the following options diagram. The first column provides an example of how to fill it in using Claire's story, the same case study as was used for the 4H Tool.

Options

	Abortion	Parenting	Adoption
My Thoughts/ Feelings	It seems like the only thing to do so that I can carry on with studies without mum or boyfriend knowing. At this stage I don't even know if the father is right for me.		
Gains	To continue University 8 Relationship that's not too heavy 4 Mum and partner need never know 5		
Losses	Open relationship that enjoyed with mum so far 5 Trust with boyfriend 5 Pregnancy - though not wanted recognise not going to be easy for me 7		
Information	Kind of abortion for stage of pregnancy		

The first row asks you to consider what it would mean to you to have an abortion, or to parent, or to consider adoption? You may have covered some of this when exploring your situation with the 4H Tool, so use that as a starting point.

Look at each choice in turn and write down your responses and the questions this raises about any of the choices.

Weighing the Gains and Losses of Each Option

Every choice we make has gains and losses, pluses and minuses, from everyday choices about what to eat, to bigger choices about where we live or work. Making one choice means that we are rejecting others. On your chart, fill in the Gains and Losses for each option.

- What would you gain from abortion and what would you lose?

- What would you would gain from parenting and what you would lose?

- What would you gain from adoption and what would you lose?

Now you have done that, look at the lists again. Some things on the list will have more weight for you than others. Underline the things on the list that carry the most weight for you – or you may want to rate them on a scale of 1–10, where 10 is the biggest or most important outcome. So, there may be 10 things to gain from one of the options and only 1 to lose, but if the loss is peace of mind, then that could be greater than all 10 gains put together. Count up the gains and losses for each option. This is a way of 'weighing' the options.

Now try to do a reality check:

- Is there anything on the lists that reflects your fears rather than reality?

- If your decision is based on your present situation, in what ways could that situation change in the future?

- If your situation changed, would you still be happy with your choice?

Making an Informed Decision

To make an informed decision, you will need to find out specific information that is relevant to your situation and the choices you are looking at.

This book contains relevant information about abortion, pregnancy and adoption, so take look at the chapters that contain the information you want to know.

Before making final choices, pause . . . Make sure you have researched everything you want to know that may be relevant to your decision. When you are ready to make your decision, go to the next chapter.

Chapter 6
Making the Choice

This chapter covers:

- Making the decision

- What happens next?

- Now what?

Making the Decision

Now is the time to look over the steps on your journey to decision and begin to plan which route you will take off the roundabout of decision. You have looked at where you are personally, explored each of the three options, thought about what each would mean for you and looked at the information you need to make a decision.

There may be people you plan to tell about your decision – friends, family, partner. Speaking it out to someone helps you to rehearse the reasons and see if you are feeling comfortable with them. Pregnancy decisions can be extremely difficult, but if you have no peace whatsoever once your decision has been made, it is an indication that the decision you have made is not sitting well with you. Regret is a difficult feeling to live with, so it is worth taking time to really think over your choice. Go back to the 4H Tool in Chapter 3 to try and find out why you are not at ease. You may want to revise your decision.

You will now also need to plan your next step, which will probably involve a visit to your doctor whatever you choose.

Remember, though, that there is continuing support whatever you choose to do: support after abortion, support with pregnancy, support with parenting, and support through and after the adoption process Support after loss may feel hard to find, but that's when you must persist until you find it and so find your way forward in life. (The chapters on parenting, adoption and abortion and the help-list at the back of the book show where help can be found).

What Happens Next?

The decision you make may or may not affect you as you expected. One of the most common emotions after making a pregnancy choice is relief, since the tension of decision-making is no longer there. For some, this feeling continues and they adjust back into life easily.

Some may have mixed feelings about what has happened and take a little time to begin to move forward with their lives. Others, however, may feel numb, angry, empty or sad, like they are grieving. We are each individual in our responses and difficult feelings can surface any time, from immediately afterwards to a long time after the event. Pregnancy counsellors do meet older women with regrets from long ago. Acknowledging these feelings, and where needed finding support to work through them, is important.

Post-abortion and post-adoption support has a focus on working through loss and on how this is processed. Grief can become complicated if our coping style is to block it or drown it out. This can happen if a loss seems too big to process or too traumatic. Even if the loss was some time ago, it is never too late to find support. Working through the loss will help us find ways of coping with emotional pain and become more resilient.

Post-adoption support is available through the local social care services, with specialised adoption counsellors trained to help. Immediate post-abortion support is available for those who want it from a few clinics and many pregnancy centres and counselling services. For those struggling after a birth, your own family and friends are vital, but the health visitor and GP can support, and so can counselling services.

For those whose abortion was some time ago and have found themselves wanting to talk about it, there are various programmes and places across the UK that can be accessed through pregnancy centres (and see Appendix 2: Finding Help, at the back of the book).

Now What?

We have explored the difficulties of making a pregnancy decision and have provided a framework for you to use to make a decision. You have travelled along the journey to decision, considering what is happening both on the outside and inside you, and the importance of looking at your responses at every level.

We now go on to explore the three choices available. Weigh them in different ways, as you have been shown: what does each mean to you personally and what do they mean in terms of gains and losses?

Part 2
Exploring Your Options

Chapter 7
Pregnancy Development Week by Week

This chapter covers:

- How the human embryo begins

- Pregnancy week by week from conception to birth

How the Human Embryo Begins

Let's look a bit more into what happens at conception – getting pregnant. Pregnancy begins in a woman's reproductive organs, see the picture below.[1]

FEMALE REPRODUCTIVE SYSTEM

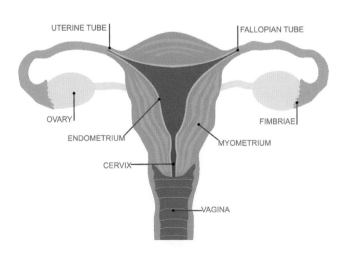

First have a look for the ovary in the picture. The ovary is where the woman makes her eggs. It is a small soft oval. Once during her monthly cycle, an egg (also called ovum) is released from one of the woman's ovaries. This egg then travels down the fallopian tube. Each egg could be fertilised for up to 2 or 3 days after she has had sex with a man or it is 'wasted' with the blood of her monthly period. From conception the embryo travels for up to a week down the fallopian tube where it is aiming to become attached (implanted) to the wall of the womb.

Conception (also called fertilization) and the beginning of pregnancy only happen if a man's sperm swims up from the vagina and reaches the egg. Vast numbers of sperm cells are released by the man during sex but usually only one will enter the woman's egg for conception. Some contraceptives such as the condom work by preventing sperm and the egg from meeting.

At conception, the genetic material of the mother and father are combined into a new gene code. This creates the brand-new blueprint of a full human being. All the information for the eye colour, sex, size and shape is packaged in a speck the size of a dot. Conception is completed in a few hours after the sperm and egg have joined and mixed their genes.

Now let's look at how tiny humans develop.

Pregnancy Week by Week from Conception to Birth

Pregnancy dates, are given in numbers of weeks from your last menstrual period (LMP), so to work out the real age of the fetus, take away two weeks from the number of weeks since your last period.

A young human is called an embryo for the first 8 weeks from conception until eight weeks old, that's 10 weeks from LMP. Then we call them a *fetus* up to birth.[2] People call their pregnancy 'the baby' at any stage of pregnancy, but this often depends on their thoughts about the future of the pregnancy at that moment.

Option: Watch the first 20 days of a fetus via this link: http://www.babycenter.com/2_inside-pregnancy-your-baby-takes-shape_10354437.bc#videoplaylist

Or https://www.youtube.com/watch?v=OD1gW88Lm-Y

Pregnancy age in weeks since your LMP (last menstrual period)	What's happening in your pregnancy?
Weeks 1–2	As we said, your pregnancy is generally dated from the first day of your LMP, because this is a date that is easy to recognise. Ovulation from the woman (egg-release) will have happened about 2 weeks later, so your partner's sperm met the egg for conception in about week 2 after your LMP (depending on the length of your menstrual cycle). Therefore, during the first two weeks, you were not actually pregnant!

A positive blood test for pregnancy can be gained as early as 4–5 days before a missed period.[3] You may see some slight implantation bleeding. This sort of bleeding or 'show' can be mistaken for a period even though you are pregnant.

This pinhead-sized one-cell embryo looks deceptively simple. Yet the cell wall of the embryo alone contains about 100,000 enzymes in working harmony. A bright *spark of light* was photographed by scientists in 2016 at the start of life, a human conception, as the man's sperm buried itself into the woman's egg. 'To see the zinc spark radiate in a burst from the human egg was breathtaking,' said Professor Teresa Woodruff.[4]

Sparks at Human Conception as the Sperm enters the Egg

(Daily Telegraph, 27 April 2016 - http://www.telegraph.co.uk/science/2016/04/26/bright-flash-of-light-marks-incredible-moment-life-begins-when-s/ reproduced with kind permission of permission Prof Teresa Woodruff, Northwestern University)

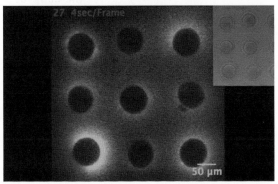

Weeks 2–3   Scientists are baffled by so much that is going on in this explosive growth.

We are near the end of Week 2 after your LMP and conception has taken place. The brand-new embryo of 1 cell carries the unique new gene code that affects every characteristic of their shape and personality for life. Within hours, hormone messages from HCG (human chorionic gonadotropin) have gone out and started to transform the body and feelings of the woman for nurturing the embryo. (Embryo means 'young one'.)

During week 3 after your LMP, the ballooning embryo is wafted along the fallopian tube towards the womb, where it implants in the wall of the womb (implantation) on day 7 of life. So, that is days 1–7 of its life so far. By the time it is one week old, the cells have multiplied 100 times from conception. Most pregnancy tests are done after this point on the HCG hormone from the embryo.

Week 4   The growing embryo (in its second week of life) divides into two: fetus and placenta. The outer cells reach out to link with the mother's blood supply and will become the placenta. Like a chick, the embryo is fed from the tiny yolk sac at this stage. Soon the placenta will take over.

Weeks 5–6   The nerve cells are already beginning to form in the brain and spinal column and sparks of activity are occurring. The basics of the major organs are in place and the heart is one of the first organs to form. The heart starts to beat at the age of 3 weeks + 5 days. Yes, the dates are that accurate! Blood is forming from the 4th week onwards.[5]

Week 6   Movements can be clearly seen on ultrasound scans once the embryo is between 4 and 6 weeks old. Little dimples on the side of the head will develop into ears, and where the eyes will be thickenings are visible.

Week 7   The developing arms and legs can be seen as small swellings (limb buds). By now the embryo is covered with a delicate layer of see-through skin.

The brain is growing rapidly, and because of this the head grows faster than the rest of the body. The inner ear has now begun to develop and the limb buds start to form cartilage, which will develop into the bones. The nervous system (the brain and spinal cord) starts to emerge.

Week 8   The embryo is the size of a jellybean by 6 weeks from conception. The legs are lengthening, though the different parts of the leg are not yet completely distinct. It will be a while before the knees, ankles, thighs and toes develop.

Week 9   The face is slowly forming. The eyes are bigger and more obvious and contain some colour. There is a mouth and tongue, complete with minute taste buds. The major internal organs such as the heart, brain, lungs, kidneys and gut are being formed and filled. All this follows the unique gene code, so every organ is unique too. Fingerprints are being engraved permanently.

Week 10   The ears are now developing on the sides of the head and the upper lip and two tiny nostrils are visible on the face. The jawbones are developing and they already contain a full set of milk teeth. The heart, now fully formed, is beating 180 times a minute. Small, jerky movements can be seen on an ultrasound scan. From this time on, the embryo is called a fetus (which means 'offspring').

Week 11   Growth spurts ahead and the bones of the face are now formed. The eyelids remain closed and won't open for a few months. The ear buds begin to resemble ears as they grow. The head makes up one-third of the fetus' length, but the body is growing fast and it is straightening. The fingers and toes are separating and fingernails appear.

55

Antenatal clinics do a dating ultra-sound scan at 11–14 weeks after LMP. The age of the fetus is given in weeks from the LMP, and from this, the midwife can give the expected date of delivery (EDD).

Week 12

The fetus, 10 weeks old, is now fully formed. All its organs, muscles, limbs and bones are in place, and the sex organs are developed. From now on, the fetus will grow and mature. Although it is moving quite a lot, it's still too early for the mother to feel those movements. The fetus pulls back from painful needles. The skeleton is made of soft cartilage which is beginning to harden into bone around this time.

Week 13

The ovaries or testes are fully developed inside the body and the genitals are forming on the outside of the body. The swelling between the legs is now developing into a penis or clitoris, although the sex of the baby cannot be seen on ultrasound scan at this stage.

Week 14

The fetus is 12 weeks old and about 10 cm from head to bottom curled up. Around this time, the fetus begins to swallow small amounts of the fluid it swims in and this is digested. The kidneys fire up and transform the swallowed fluid into urine, which passes back into the amniotic fluid.

Week 15

At this stage, the fetus will be starting to hear and it may be able to hear its mother's voice, heartbeat and sounds from her digestive system, as well as muted sounds from the world outside. The eyes also start to become sensitive to light; they are closed, but may sense a bright light from outside shone through the tummy.

Week 16

The fetus is beginning to make some facial expressions. The nervous system makes the arms and legs flex. About now, the hands can reach and hold each other and can form a fist.

Weeks 17-19   The fetus is growing bigger and the head and body are more in proportion. The face begins to look much more human, with eyebrows and eyelashes beginning to develop. The eyes can move now, although the eyelids remain closed. The mouth can now open and close. The lines on the skin of the fingers are now established, which means that the fetus already has his or her own individual fingerprints. The fetus is moving around quite a bit at this stage, and may respond to music or other loud noises from the outside world.

In UK, the NHS offers a high-definition scan between 18 and 21 weeks. That is an ultrasound scan of the body. Even though great care is taken, practitioners can sometimes reassure that all is well when it is not or mistakenly advise that something is wrong.

Babies born from this stage on may survive with breathing movements for some hours, but even with intensive care, they cannot live long.

Weeks 20-24   Around this time, the fetus becomes covered in a very fine, soft hair and is beginning to get into a pattern of sleeping and waking, which may not be the same as the mother's. The lungs are not yet able to function properly, but the fetus is practising breathing actions. Oxygen supplies come from the mother's placenta until birth.

Premature babies born as early as 22 weeks weighing just 1 lb or ½ kg, now have a reasonable chance of survival with intensive care. However, while survival is certainly possible, there is a significant risk of long-term disability. (See the Chapter 21 'Premature Birth After Abortion' for more information). A baby born at 24 weeks from the LMP has a far better chance of a healthy future than at 22 weeks.

As a doctor working with new-borns in intensive care, I was happy if a baby stayed inside mum until they were at least 28 weeks, because I knew that baby would usually romp through life outside Mum from 28 or 30 weeks. (Recent evidence suggests that even babies born at 34–37 weeks have a risk of early and long-term complications.)[6]

Weeks 25-28   The fetus now moves around a lot and reacts to sound and touch. The eyelids open for the first time and soon will start blinking. The brain, lungs and digestive system are completely formed now but need time to become fully functional. By 28 weeks the fetus is perfectly formed.

Weeks 29-32   The fetus moves around more and more. The skin becomes less wrinkled as they put on weight. The fetus is sucking their thumb or finger and their eyes can focus on objects.

Weeks 33-36   The fetus' bones continue to harden, apart from the skull bones which will remain separated and soft until after birth. At 33 weeks, the brain and nervous system are completely developed, and at 36 weeks the lungs are fully formed.

Weeks 37-birth   The pregnancy is called full-term at 37 weeks from the LMP. All being well, the fetus' head moves down into the pelvis about now, beginning their journey of birth. The average British baby weighs 7 lbs 8 oz at birth.

Reassurance

Most women manage pregnancy and deliver their baby fine, despite the big changes that pregnancy brings. Premature babies can live from 22 weeks onwards, and though risky for the baby, they can do well with expert care.

Does the fetus feel pain at abortion?

This is relevant to you if you are considering a mid-term or late abortion, because you may not be offered pain relief for the fetus. The anaesthetic for the woman may not numb the fetus much against pain,[7] so you may wish to discuss the following with your anaesthetist.

What to discuss with your anaesthetist before abortion

You need to know that debate continues on at what stage the fetus can feel pain. So the following may help you discuss a more humane end to the life of your fetus with the doctors involved.

Videos show the fetus pulling back from needles from around 12 weeks old. The view of current scientific opinion is that a fetus can *feel* pain like you or me from between 20 and 24 weeks,[8] but some say 15 weeks.[9] So we see that in the case of surgery *to help the fetus live*, which is done in the womb from about 18 weeks, anaesthesia is used. This shows that doctors do have concerns that fetuses may be feeling pain earlier than 20 weeks.

The method of abortion used by the NHS for late abortions begins with an injection of potassium chloride to stop the fetal heart beating. Some anaesthetists have recommended prior injection of a muscle-paralysing drug, presumably to stop the fetus jumping as the painful potassium takes effect. A jumping fetus might be felt by the mother and might evade the needle of the surgeon or anaesthetist. The fetus is then delivered by induction of labour or surgical destruction and removal through the vagina. This is especially used for older and larger fetuses from 16 weeks onwards.[10]

British gynaecologists and anaesthetists now usually administer fentanyl – a powerful painkiller – directly to the fetus immediately prior to the lethal injection, but it is not yet standard policy and it is unclear from what fetal age this procedure is used. Be sure to ask for it if you want to.

Fetal pain laws in some states of the USA now enforce mandatory administration of fetal pain relief prior to the abortion from 20 weeks onwards.

There were 225 known abortions reported at 24 weeks or older in the UK in 2016. These were for reasons such as Down's syndrome, malformation, spina bifida, cerebral palsy and cleft palate.[11]

Chapter 8
Parenting Explored

This chapter covers:

- My circumstances now

- Can I cope?

- What help is available to me?

- What next?

Evelyn's story

When my GP gave me the news that I was over 14 weeks pregnant, I couldn't sleep. Yes, I had missed some periods recently, but I explained them away with change of country and stress.

My mind was full of thoughts. How could I miss the early days of my pregnancy? What was happening to my body? How could I adapt to the idea of becoming a mum? I knew it would change my life forever.

I found my partner Pete and asked him: Would I be able to look after my baby in good times and in bad? What if things were not all normal with the baby? What if I couldn't cope? What about my job and my plans for a career? Was he ready to start a family? Would we both be willing to give up our freedom, our peaceful nights and our energy?

I was overwhelmed. I felt weak and quite sick at the sheer thought of it all.

This story shows the shock that an unplanned pregnancy can bring and highlights some of the issues involved when thinking about parenting. It may be difficult, for a number of reasons, to think about continuing the pregnancy and having a baby. This chapter helps you look at this option realistically.

My Circumstances Now

Often there are no easy answers to the situation you are in. Below are some common situations:

• It's to do with the father

It may be that you don't want to go on to parent because you don't want to be connected to the person who is the father of the baby. He may be abusive, or you just don't want to be with him, or you can't be with him (he may already be with someone else). It can be helpful to try to separate out the two decisions you're faced with:

1. Is it to do with going on with the man? The answer to this may be a clear 'no' or it may be, 'I would if I could' and carry some heartache with it. Coming to terms with what your future relationship with the father may be is important.

2. Is it about having the baby? Am I able to love and care for this child on my own? Is there a way it could work? Is it possible to break the relationship and continue the pregnancy? What do I need to consider?

• It's to do with other people knowing

It may be that you don't want to continue the pregnancy because there is someone who you feel cannot know about it. This could be your parent(s), school, work, community, or your partner especially if the pregnancy is from someone else.

Often these situations need looking at on an individual basis with a trained counsellor, to help you explore how to move forward. Keeping a secret like this can be overwhelming, totally absorbing and exhausting. Being able to share it with someone outside your situation may be the most helpful way of thinking it through.

• Something may be wrong with the baby

It may be that you are feeling you cannot continue parenting because there is a risk that your baby may have a disability. You may have been excited to be pregnant and looking forward to having a baby but some recent test result or worries about medication you have taken may be causing you concern.

You can check out the effects of any medication on the developing fetus by looking online at www.medicines.org.uk, and you could talk through the implications of this with a professional. No one can give assurances that your baby will be born perfect, and 'disability' can cover a very wide range of issues, from very mild problems like cleft palate to major problems like spina bifida.

Exploring exactly what you have been told, how accurate a diagnosis you have, and all the fears that come with that, is the next step. Any mention of disability in the fetus can bring on panic, so it is important to have time and space to think through any implications before making a decision. (More on this comes in Chapter 15, 'Antenatal Screening and Fetal Disability'.)

• It's to do with the timing
It may be that you are feeling like this is the wrong time for you to have a baby: you may be still studying; you may have just started a job or just got a promotion; you may already have the number of children you want; you may feel like you have not had chance to do the things you want to do. There is a cost to parenting that you are counting – physically, emotionally, financially, as well as in time and commitment. You will need to weigh up whether the things you would be sacrificing now can be picked up later, or whether you could continue to do those things with a child.

Can I Cope?
At this point, I suggest you go back to your notes from the 'Making Choices' chapters. Look back at your gains and losses for parenting and how you rated them. If you did not complete that exercise, do it now.

Go back to the 4H Tool and look again at what you are bringing into the situation. Ask yourself:

• What internal resources and strengths do I have?
What personal qualities do I have that would help me to parent? What personal qualities might stop me parenting well? Is there anything I could put in place to help me if I'm struggling?

- **What external support do I have?**

Parents/friends/partner? Are there any agencies out there that could support me if I decide to continue the pregnancy? How could they help?

Whilst parenting can bring much love and joy into your life, there are also challenges. Raising a child can put pressure on your finances, your time and on your relationships, and it can affect your own freedom and your work or studies.

Depending on what your circumstances are, you may be able to find information from your local council, health services, government services or organisations like Citizens Advice. If you have a pregnancy centre in your area, they may be able to help you with the information you need and provide you with practical support. Alternatively, you may want to use the internet to find out information, and there are some websites below that you may find useful.

What Help is Available to Me?

Look for what help may be available to you in your specific situation. Knowing what support is there for you is especially important if lack of support is a main reason for not wanting to parent. If it seems overwhelming, ask a pregnancy centre or one of the other agencies mentioned to help you:

- **Finances**

Visit https://www.gov.uk for information about cash benefits you can claim when you are pregnant or have a child.

There is information for asylum seekers at https://www.gov.uk/asylum-support/what-youll-get.

Students can visit http://www.nhs.uk/conditions/pregnancy-and-baby/pages/maternity-paternity-leave-benefits.aspx

Help for non-English speakers is usually available.

- **Healthcare**

Once you have registered with a local GP in the UK, you are entitled to free prenatal and antenatal health care (https://www.maternityaction.org.uk/ explains entitlement for asylum seekers).

• **Housing**

If you have housing needs, you can contact the Housing Department of your local council for housing advice. See also Shelter (http://england. shelter.org.uk) and Life (https://lifecharity.org.uk).

• **Education**

It may be possible to continue your pregnancy and your education. If you are under 16, the local authority has a legal requirement to provide you with education. How this happens varies across regions and schools. For more information go to: https://www.babycentre.co.uk/x1043670/ im-school-age-and-pregnant-can-i-keep-my-education-going.

If you are a student under 20, you may be eligible for childcare costs under 'Care to Learn'. Check out these websites:

https://www.gov.uk/care-to-learn/overview

https://www.nus.org.uk/en/news/information-for-student-parents/

• **Single parents**

Support is available through Gingerbread www.gingerbread.org.uk and, if you are having problems with isolation, through Home-Start http:// www.home-start.org.uk.

The local pregnancy centre or LIFE may also be able to offer you baby clothes and equipment, as well as emotional support throughout your pregnancy.

What Next?

Now that you've had a chance to consider some of the issues around having a baby, spend some time imagining yourself as a mum and note any emotions and concerns before making any firm decisions.

Chapter 9
Adoption Explored

This chapter covers:

- Why think about adoption?

- What happens in adoption?

- Special guardianship

- Regrets after adoption?

- What contact can I have?

- What now?

Why Think About Adoption?

Thinking about giving your baby for adoption in our society takes courage, since it is much misunderstood. However, there are circumstances where adoption can be a loving choice. Here are just a few:

- The baby could be in danger from others through staying with the parent.

- The mother doesn't agree with abortion but recognises she cannot parent given her circumstances.

- The mother chooses what she considers to be a 'better life' for her child.

- The mother risks rejection from her community as a single parent.

It is important to think through 3 different options:

1. Fostering

2. Special guardianship

3. Adoption

For those who are considering adoption but are still uncertain, there is the possibility of voluntary foster care while you think it over.

Special guardianship is a longer-term option, until the child is 18 at least – but the mother can often have contact. Usually the Local Authority is involved with all these decisions.

For adoption, you can also choose to go to an independent adoption agency (addresses at the end of this chapter and at the back of the book). Some parents want to keep their baby but the local social authority does not feel it is safe for the child, and this leads to 'enforced adoption'. However, the focus of this chapter is with those who are considering adoption as a choice.

> 'Adoption is a brave, generous decision that will bring joy to adopters and give the child a chance of life.'
>
> Dr Kirsty Saunders, MBChB, DCH, Adoption Paediatrician

Adoption provides a child with a permanent new family and home when living with their biological family is not possible.

> Dominic has fetal alcohol syndrome which can impair mental function. His adoptive parents Ron and Avril say, 'Since adopting Dominic, he is just so happy, always happy. Dominic is very intelligent. You can feel quite chuffed you have given a child a chance of life that maybe they wouldn't have had.' Watch at: http://corambaaf.org.uk/res/videos

The numbers[1]

- As of 31 March 2016, 3,540 children under one-year old were being looked after in care in England, while 230 were adopted before they were a year old.

- As of 31 March 2016, 3,350 approved adoptive parents were waiting to be matched with children.

What Happens in Adoption?

There are many people who want to adopt a baby and have been through a rigorous screening process, which means that it should be possible to find a home for your child. You will be able to discuss what kind of family you want your child to be placed in.

Preparations for the adoption can begin before your child is born, but no permanent arrangements will be made until after you have given birth. Even then, you will be completely free to change your mind. However, once an adoption order has been made (when your child has been with their new family for a minimum of ten weeks) it cannot be changed.

The process has four stages. There is plenty of time for you to rethink and change your mind.

1. A social worker will talk to you about adoption and provide initial counselling. You can request the kind of parents you would like for your baby. Agencies try to place your baby with adopting parents of your preferred ethnicity but there is an ongoing shortage of minority families seeking to adopt. There is a rise in interracial adoption.[2]

2. Immediately after the birth, you can spend some time with the baby if you want to. If you are very likely to want adoption, the baby would be placed with adopters from the beginning, but you can still see the baby and still change your mind. The baby will be placed with foster parents for at least six weeks, during which time you can visit.

3. The baby is then placed with the adoptive parents and, after three months, the adoption order will be applied for.

4. You will then be asked by the social worker to sign a legal document and the court will make an adoption order. You are not required to attend court, but after this point you cannot change your mind.

The Adoption and Children Act 2002 (England and Wales), which came into force in September 2005, brought about several changes to adoption. Some of these changes affect the process of adoption:

- The Local Authority for social care is now obliged to first investigate the family of the birth mother to see if anyone is suitable to adopt the child.

- They will also look at the family of the birth father, if he has been identified. If the birth mother objects strongly, her reasons for objection will be investigated. However, the father only has a say in the decision if he has parental responsibility (that means he is named on the birth certificate or you are married).

Special Guardianship
Special Guardianship Order means that the birth mother can select someone who is willing to be a guardian to her baby (usually someone in the family). Parental responsibility is then shared between the birth parent and the special guardian until the child is 18 or over, but the special guardian is the senior partner, so can decide education, health and residence issues. The order is a private law provision, so the guardian must apply to court for an order to be made. This would normally need the help of a solicitor. The local authority is then asked by the court to send a social worker to assess the situation and compile a 'suitability report'.

Regrets After Adoption?
During my four decades as a medical professional, I was humbled by the courage and willingness of mothers with an unwanted pregnancy to give their child for adoption. I cannot remember any with serious regrets, but this is not to say it never happens. John McKeegan, who was adopted at birth, writes, 'With my involvement in adoption groups I can tell you, yes, there are relinquishing [giving away] parents who later regret giving up their child.'[3]

'Our adopted daughter gave us hell for the first thirteen years. Then she changed into a wonderful person. Recently I saw a picture of her wedding with her birth mother standing beside her. (It was illness that prevented me from attending.)' – Mrs X

The birth mother is always encouraged to write a letter to be read when the child is older, so that the mother or couple can explain to the child why they had to take this step. Usually there is a photo of Mum with the baby for him or her to see later.

John's mother gave birth to him in South America and he now lives in Europe. She says, 'Knowing he was well has helped to heal the wounds.'

She could accept the decision and solution. She keeps contact via a trusted contact person. John sends his birth mum a picture every birthday to show how he is doing.

John says, 'I did find it strange to find I had parents from South America and it was emotional to meet my mum, but well worth it.'

What Contact Can I Have?

You will have opportunity to prepare a 'Life Story' book with photos that will be shared with your child by the adoptive parents and there is almost always an opportunity for letter-box contact at a specified time every year, which happens through the adoption agency or through the local authority. This means that you will receive an update on your child's progress and you can respond by placing a letter on file which may or may not be shared with the child, but is there should the child want to look when they are 18. If you want future contact with the child, you must register an interest in being found.

One adoption professional says she knows of several adoptions of babies from birth, who later have good relationships with their birth parents. Also, it can end up where the birth parent and adopting parents have a good relationship, like an extended family.[4]

What Now?

If you decide that the right choice for you and your baby is adoption, you have nothing to be ashamed of – it can be a very loving option. You are entitled to counselling throughout the procedure and afterwards, to work through all the different emotions you will have. Local authorities are good at providing this if the mother wants it.

Choosing adoption is a viable option for your baby's future – full of hope and potential – but, as with all pregnancy decisions, there are emotions attached to the choice you make. If you are considering adoption, get as much expert advice as possible. There are many experienced people who are willing to support you.

Talk to family and trusted friends privately about your thoughts on this subject. You have time to consider adoption. Rushing will not help your decision, so use this time wisely so that you make a decision which will give you peace of mind for now as well as for the long term.

For more information on adoption, see 'Appendix 2: Finding Help' at the back of the book.

Chapter 10
Abortion Explored

This chapter covers:

- Basic information

- How abortions are done

- Abortions at different stages of pregnancy

- Abortion risks and after-effects

Basic Information

Abortion is a significant medical procedure. The woman – or couple – first needs to fully understand all the implications. This information tends to help ownership of the choice by the woman.

Abortion is the removal of a pregnancy from the womb of a woman before natural birth. It can be referred to by professionals as 'induced abortion', TOP (termination of pregnancy), STOP (suction termination of pregnancy) or EMA (early medical abortion) depending on the stage of pregnancy and method used.

Miscarriage, also called 'spontaneous abortion', is the natural loss of the pregnancy before birth. In most cases, the cause is unknown.

Abortions in the UK are usually carried out legally up to 24 weeks from the LMP (last menstrual period), though most are done before 12 weeks. It is possible to have an abortion up to term (birth due date) in exceptional circumstances. Most abortions take place in private clinics, paid for by the NHS. Some are done in NHS hospitals. You may be seen by your GP and/or at a clinic. Two doctors are meant to agree that there are legal grounds for abortion, and recently there have been nurse-led abortions, with public comments raised about safety.

Home abortions, using drugs obtained online, are risky and you are advised not to attempt this for your own safety.

How Abortions are Done

There are two ways of having an abortion:

- Medically, using tablets (now over half of all UK abortions).

- Surgically, involving an operation under sedation or anaesthetic (local or general).

The details of what happens depends on the stage of pregnancy.

Before abortion, you are entitled to

- Spoken and written information to help you decide, including counselling.

- Tests for your blood group and sexually transmitted infections (including Chlamydia).

- Written details of all possible side effects.

- You may be offered a scan and a smear. The scan is to show the age of the fetus. Clinics may not show you the scan in case it moves your feelings or prompts a change of choice. Some pregnancy counsellors offer a scan as information for holistic choice making.

You can change your mind at any time. Information and support should be offered if you decide not to have an abortion.[1]

Abortion at Different Stages of Pregnancy
Medical abortions

- **EMA (early medical abortion) up to 9 weeks:** EMAs involve two visits to the hospital or clinic following initial assessment. The first visit is to

Abortion methods at different dates of pregnancy.

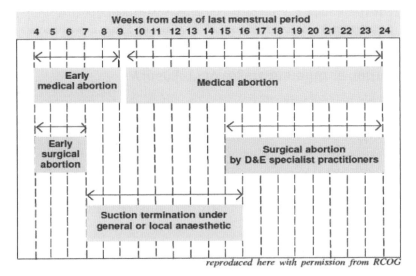

reproduced here with permission from RCOG

take the abortion pill (mifepristone). This blocks the hormones that help the pregnancy to continue. Bleeding may continue over a week.

• At the second visit, around 1–3 days later, a dose of prostaglandin (misoprostol) is given either by mouth or in the vagina. This usually causes the womb to expel the pregnancy, with the fetus, placenta and blood, within four to six hours. It is possible to go home on the same day, even if the abortion is not completed. In this case, a follow-up appointment would be needed to confirm the pregnancy has ended.

• **Over 9 weeks:** Medical abortion may involve a stay at the hospital or clinic at the second visit until the abortion is complete, and may need more than one dose of prostaglandin and additional pain relief.

RED FLAG

Medical Abortion

A medical abortion may be risky in certain circumstances: allergy to any of the abortion drugs; taking blood-clotting, anti-inflammatory or corticosteroid medication; suffering from medical conditions such as of the liver or kidney.

Surgical abortions

- **Suction aspiration under 7 weeks:** This is done in the same way as a suction termination (below), but a manual syringe (rather than a machine) may be used under conscious sedation to remove the pregnancy. Failure may mean that additional surgery is needed.

- **Suction termination 7–15 weeks:** This is the most common way surgical abortions are carried out and they take place either under general anaesthetic or under local anaesthetic, conscious but sedated. The neck of the womb (the cervix), which is normally tightly shut through pregnancy, is gradually stretched using dilators until it is wide enough for the pregnancy to be removed with a large suction tube. The cervix may be softened beforehand using vaginal pessaries (misoprostol).

- **D & E (dilatation and evacuation) from about 15 weeks:** The cervix is gradually stretched and opened (dilated) and the pregnancy is removed with a suction tube and forceps. It is done under general anaesthetic. An ultrasound scan is advised at the same time to try to reduce side effects and ensure that the procedure is completed.

- **Late abortions (over 20 weeks)** can be done by medical or surgical means. Medically, the procedure imitates induction of labour and delivery. This includes 'therapeutic abortion', where a pregnancy is ended because of a fetal disability.

Sometimes an injection is given into the heart of the fetus to stop it before abortion takes place.

Surgery can be carried out either through the vagina or by Caesarean section (C-section) through a cut in the skin of the abdomen – which route depends on several factors, including the age of the pregnancy.

Abortion Risks and After-effects

In this section, we list just the main after-effects in two groups: firstly, the early after-effects, which are likely to occur the first couple of weeks, and secondly, the longer-term ones which can occur from two weeks after an abortion, up to decades later. We cover the after-effects in more detail in Chapter 12 'Overview of the After-effects of Abortion'.

In 2009 it was reported that medical abortion has *4 times more* adverse effects in the six weeks afterwards than surgical abortion.[2]

After-effects in the first two weeks following abortion:[3]

- **Infection** of the reproductive organs can follow either medical or surgical abortion, especially when a sexually transmitted infection (STI) is already present. The Royal College of Obstetricians and Gynaecologists reports, 'infective complications occur in 10% of women' at abortion.[4] Infection is less likely to occur if a woman is taking antibiotics at the time of the procedure, but they do not always work. Infection can result in pelvic inflammatory disease (PID) which can cause tubal blockage and so may affect a woman's fertility. (There is further information on this in Chapter 20 'Infertility After Abortion'. For more on PID, a helpful diagram and notes can be found at http://www.patient.co.uk/health/pelvic-inflammatory-disease-leaflet.)

- **Pain** during and after medical or surgical abortion is common. It can range from abdominal discomfort to intense pain. It was rated 'as bad as it can be' by 1 in 4 British women who'd had an abortion in an Aberdeen study.[5] In the United States it was reported that as many as 1 in 2 women who'd had a medical abortion with drugs considered their abdominal pain was 'severe'.[6] (See more in Chapter 16 'Physical After-effects of Abortion'.)

- **Pain felt by the fetus** is possible in mid-term or late abortions (see the end of Chapter 7 'Pregnancy Development Week by Week').

- **Incomplete abortion** means failure to remove all the fetal parts and placenta. This happens in fewer than 1 in 100 cases, in both medical and surgical abortions.[7] When this occurs, further surgery is required.

- **Excessive vaginal bleeding** at the time of the abortion resulting in the need for a blood transfusion. This happens in around 1 in 1,000 cases. This increases to 4 in 1,000 cases for termination of pregnancies that are beyond 20 weeks.[8]

- **Damage to the cervix** (neck of the womb) at the time of the procedure. This happens in up to 1 in every 100 surgical abortions. This is less likely when performed by experienced clinicians, however, experienced surgeons are not always available in the UK.[9] Damage to the womb and reproductive organs can lead to infertility. Estimates range from between 1 to 15 women out of 1,000.[10]

- **Failed abortion** can mean the **fetus survives** the abortion attempts and is born alive. In 2008, 66 fetuses were born alive this way and year by year some survive to grow up and speak of their feelings about their parent.[11] (More on this can be found in Chapter 16 'Physical After-effects of Abortion'.)

RED FLAG

After Abortion

Contact a doctor early in case of the following:

- Vaginal bleeding that soaks more than two sanitary pads within two consecutive hours.

- Feeling faint, as this can be a sign of internal bleeding.

- Temperature greater than 38°C, can mean infection is getting a grip.

- Abdominal pain.

- Nausea, vomiting, or diarrhoea that continues for more than 24 hours

- Still feeling pregnant one or two weeks after the procedure. This can mean a failed abortion and the fetus is still alive in the womb.

Long-term risks

There has been much debate around the long-term risks of abortion. Beware of claims that risks are either minimal on one hand or massive on the other. This essential section summarises some of the opinions so you can make up your own mind. (More detail can be found in Chapter 12 'Overview of the After-effects of Abortion' and in Part 3).[12]

- **Future preterm birth.** A study combining 37 other studies found that one abortion made a preterm birth in the follow-on pregnancy 27% more likely. Two or more abortions made preterm birth 62% more likely (see Chapter 21 'Premature Birth After Abortion'.[13]

- **Breast cancer abortion link?** The question of whether abortion leads to a higher risk of breast cancer in later life is much debated. For this reason, Chapter 18 is devoted to the issue in Part 3 of this book. In brief, research says that for a young woman who has never been pregnant, any factor that delays her first full-term pregnancy (FFTP) will bring a higher risk of breast cancer for her later on. And abortion is a factor that often delays FFTP, so there is one major risk. This means that for every five years' delay in FFTP there is a link with nearly a 20% increase in risk of breast cancer, for a woman up to the age of 35.[14]

- **Miscarriages and premature birth.** In subsequent pregnancies, miscarriages and premature birth have been linked with damage to the cervix during abortion (1 in 100 women), as mentioned above. (More in on this in Chapter 20 'Infertility after Abortion'.)

- **Fertility concerns after abortion.** This debate can be captured by a snapshot from two views:

The Royal College of Obstetricians and Gynaecologists (RCOG) stated in 2011 that 'Published studies strongly suggest that infertility is not a consequence of *uncomplicated* induced abortion.'[15] But beware that word 'uncomplicated', because the College admits 'complications' (after-effects from abortion) occur often. For instance, infections occurring from 1 in 10 abortions *are* a threat to future fertility. The College admits, 'Post-abortion infection may later result in tubal infertility.'[16]

Meanwhile, researchers in North America, after 10 years studying the evidence, concluded in 2013 that 'Evidence linking *infertility* to previous induced abortion is *overwhelming*.'[17] More on this follows in Chapter 20 'Infertility After Abortion'. At the end of the day, it's your choice who you believe and your health at stake.

- **Repeat abortions** bring higher risks than one abortion, not only for breast cancer but also premature birth in subsequent pregnancies. (Read more on repeat abortions in Chapter 12 'Overview of the After-effects of Abortion' and Chapter 20 'Infertility After Abortion'.)

- **Mental health problems after abortion.**

Counsellors and other carers have reported both short-term and long-term effects to mental health after abortion for decades. Research suggests that having an unwanted pregnancy is already a red flag for mental and emotional ill health, whether the woman continues with the pregnancy or has an abortion. This is to be expected, as for any major stress factor in life.

Recent studies suggest links with small to moderate increases in major mental health problems like depression, anxiety and suicidal thoughts which may occur after abortion, even in women with no previous history of problems.[18],[19]

Previous history of mental or emotional ill health is a red flag of caution before option for an abortion, because it seems to be more likely to trigger post-abortion emotional problems.[20] A pre-abortion checklist to help predict the likelihood of severe post-abortion emotional trouble can be found in Chapter 19 'Mental and Emotional Effects of Pregnancy Loss'.

• Mortality after abortion

Thankfully, death *during* abortion appears to be rare if there is good medical care. However, there is compelling evidence that abortion can contribute to the deaths of young women, both in the first year and the first decade following an abortion. This evidence is from excellent record linkage studies undertaken in Finland, Denmark,[21] Wales[22] and California. A significant portion of these extra deaths are due to suicide, accident and murder, which may indicate elevated levels of self-destructive or risk-taking behaviours. It does not mean abortion is the *direct and immediate* cause of these deaths, but there is strong evidence that it is a *contributing factor.*

The basic messages to guide decisions are:

1. A woman's risk of dying in the year after an abortion is about three times higher than the risk of dying in the year following childbirth. Mika Gissler (in 2004) showed that the mortality rate for every 100,000 women (adjusted for the woman's age) in one year was 26 for pregnancy or birth, 82 for women who'd had an abortion in the previous year and 56 for miscarriage loss or ectopic loss.[23]

2. The women's average age of death linked with abortion was about 28 years.[24]

3. This elevated rate of death following abortion appears within 180 days and continues for 10 or more years.[25]

4. Repeat abortions do matter: one abortion increases the risk of a woman's early death by about 50%, two abortions by 100%, and three abortions by 150 %.[26]

5. It's a long-term risk and the years of risk stack up. A study of low-income Californian women over an 8-year period following their abortions reported about 300 extra deaths per 100,000 women (compared to women who gave birth) with an average age at death of 28 years.[27],[28] To imagine 100,000 women think of Wembley Stadium in London filled up – there would be quite a gap if 300 of them died from an avoidable cause.

6. In contrast, giving birth reduces the risk of women's death, compared to the increased risk of death associated with abortion. Women who gave birth to two or three pregnancies at full term have about half the risk of death compared to those who have never been pregnant.[29] So, pregnancy and giving birth appears to be better for a woman's health than never being pregnant and is many times safer again than having an abortion.

There is much more information on this in Chapter 17 'Mortality of Women After Birth and Abortion'.

Grieving and disposal of your fetus

In England and Wales, the fetus should be disposed of according to your wishes, whether incineration, cremation or burial. You may need to ask and insist on your wishes being carried out, as reports persist of fetuses being disposed of in general hospital incinerators. Advice is given about what your options are if you are to lose your pregnancy at home (such as during medical abortion). In Scotland, the options are either cremation or burial, not incineration.[30]

Some women and couples prefer to go through a proper burial of their remains, sometimes with a religious ceremony. If you came from abroad for an abortion, you should be able to take home the remains in an opaque container.

More advice for those grieving after abortion due to fetal disability can be found in Chapter 15 'Antenatal Screening and Disability in the Fetus'. Another reason linked to this, but very rare, is abortion due to illness in the mother. Appendix 2 'Finding Help' at the back of the book may help you.

Some people have found that the process of grieving and healing can be helped by the planting of a memorial such as a tree in a special place. The question of whether to tell the siblings of the deceased is very personal, but many have found it very helpful; siblings and relatives will probably come to know of it one day, and will have their own sense of loss and grief.

Abortion after-care

It is considered normal for a woman to bleed from the vagina after the procedure, for nine to ten days on average, though it can last longer.

Before leaving the clinic, the woman will be given information about pain management, vaginal bleeding and the loss via the vagina of further parts of the fetus and placenta. Written advice about looking out for possible after-effects and who to contact should they occur should be provided before leaving the clinic.

Chapter 11
Abortion Law in the UK and Abroad

This chapter covers:

- Informed consent

- Law for those under 16 years old

- Men and the abortion law

- When is abortion legal?

- What you can expect from your doctor

- The law in Northern Ireland, the Isle of Man and the Channel Islands

- Abortion law in the USA, Canada and Australia

The key thing to know – wherever you are in the world and whatever the abortion law says – is this: your health professionals have a duty to protect your health and not to harm you, your family and future children in any advice or treatment they give.

It's because abortion can adversely affect you, your family, and children not yet conceived, that you yourself should know your medical risks and lawful rights. This is needed, since abortion goes ahead in the UK and many parts of the world with little restraint, and at times outright pressure to abort. This pressure can come from professionals and others – so you leave the choice to others at your own risk.

Knowing the truth will help set you free, and empower your free, personal and informed choice.

This chapter includes the points about British abortion law relevant to your safety before, during and after choosing abortion. Most of these apply to those living in England, Scotland and Wales. Northern Ireland and the Isle of Man, other offshore islands and some other countries are mentioned here also.

The abortion law for England, Wales and Scotland was created over the last fifty years to help people make difficult moral and clinical decisions on pregnancy. It was created to protect you and your pregnancy from bad medical practice. It also protects doctors who are doing their best in a complicated and difficult area. However, a widely held belief is that the UK law is failing; it is a broken safety net full of holes, so you need to know where you are vulnerable to its abuse.

Informed Consent

Informed consent is about you being able to trust your professionals to give you all the information you need along with a deep respect for your right to decide for yourself. The UK law does not grant abortion on demand though in practice that is what we have.

A landmark legal case in 2015 changed your consent rights.[1] You can now expect in writing, full and complete information from the professionals, as well as shared decision-making with them. Doctors who ignore or withhold information, even about a small risk, may be breaking the law. Both doctor and patient are legally bound to refuse abortion unless the legal criteria are met.

- You should expect full information on your three options: parenting, adoption and abortion. Women's views should be respected when they do not wish to know these options.[2]

- Before you must decide, you should expect information which is impartial, accurate and evidence-based on all possible physical, emotional and social risks and implications.

- Information should be both spoken and written.[3]

- Every woman who requests an abortion should be offered the opportunity to discuss her options and choices with a trained pregnancy counsellor at every stage of the care pathway.[4]

While most doctors aim to be neutral, some professionals have been overprotective, telling teens and women what they should do. For example, recently a 16-year-old pregnant girl who had made clear she wanted to have the baby, backed by her parents promising practical support, was very upset to still be pressurised by two GPs and a nurse towards abortion.[5]

Abortion to get a boy or a girl?
Abortion on the grounds of choosing the sex of the baby is not lawful.[6]

Law for Those Under 16 Years Old
The law protects the confidentiality of a person under 16. It allows a young person under the age of 16 to give her own consent to be given reproductive health advice and treatment without parental knowledge or consent, if certain criteria apply and the treatment is in her best interests. However, everything possible should be done to involve the parents if possible.

Men and the Abortion Law
Legally, men as the father of the fetus have no say in an abortion decision. The weight of decision-making rests with the woman. This may be a reason why many men are passive in the decision-making process. Further information about the roles of men and the effects on men can be found in Chapter 14 'Men, Pregnancy and Abortion'.

When is Abortion Legal?
Abortion is legal if it can be justified under the UK Abortion Act 1967. The Act looks at the health of the pregnant woman in her mind and body, the wellbeing of the fetus and the wellbeing of existing children. The law does not allow abortion 'on demand'.

Just as pregnant women have different views on the future of their fetus, doctors have different opinions on how to interpret the law. This explains why you may be refused an abortion but your friend in a similar situation, seeing different professionals, may be offered an abortion. Furthermore doctors, like patients, have their own consciences to follow – one doctor's conscience may say it is right that a woman can demand an abortion, another's may say it is right that the fetus and woman should be protected, and that the law is there to protect both.

The Abortion Act 1967 (amended in 1990) gives the following legal grounds for abortion in England and Wales. But note, it does not protect subsequent children who may be damaged by premature birth as an aftereffect of previous abortion:

1. **(a)** That the pregnancy has not exceeded its twenty-fourth (24th) week and that the continuance of the pregnancy would involve risk, greater than if the pregnancy were terminated, of injury to the physical or mental health of the pregnant woman or any existing children of her family [up to 24 weeks];

   (b) the termination is necessary to prevent grave permanent injury to the physical or mental health of the pregnant woman [no time-limit, so up to 40 weeks];

   (c) that the continuance of the pregnancy would involve risk to the life of the pregnant woman, greater than if the pregnancy were terminated [no time limit, so up to 40 weeks]; or

   (d) the continuance of the pregnancy would involve risk, greater than if the pregnancy were terminated, of injury to the physical or mental health of any existing child(ren) of the family of the pregnant woman [up to 24 weeks];

   (e) that there is a substantial risk that if the child were born it would suffer from such physical or mental abnormalities as to be seriously handicapped [no time limit, so up to birth].

Most legal abortions in England and Wales are carried out to bring *lower* risk of injury to the *mental health* of the woman than a baby might bring; which is Ground 1(a) in the Abortion Act. You can see above that the key condition to be fulfilled is 'risk, greater than if the pregnancy were terminated, of injury to the physical or mental health of the pregnant woman'. The problem is the growing evidence – known for years – that abortion adds its own mental health risks *greater* than if the pregnancy went to birth. This book should help you weigh up these risks for yourself (see Chapters 10 'Abortion Explored' and 12 'Overview of After-effects of Abortion').

The Abortion Act also says that two 'medical practitioners' must sign for each abortion under one of the legal grounds (the rare exception to this is in a medical emergency to save the life of the mother). However, there are currently cases of the abortion pill being administered by nurse practitioners alone, because of a loophole in the law. Expert doctors have severely criticised the safety and legality of nurse led abortions.

What You Can Expect From Your Doctor

Under this special law, two doctors, acting with all the trust and good faith that their position demands, must be satisfied that you are fully informed of material risks in your particular case. The law says they must decide whether a person in your position would find those risks significant.

In order to do this, they must understand your thoughts, your feelings and your beliefs, and what stage of pregnancy you are at. This puts a duty on professionals to see you in person and if necessary examine you, often on more than one occasion. Beware the clinics and doctors uncovered who have been pre-signing bunches of abortion forms without seeing you.

Your right to a second opinion

Here are some scenarios where you might find you need a second opinion:

- **Duty of a doctor to offer a second opinion.** In the community, if a woman sees a doctor who feels there are not sufficient grounds for abortion, then she can ask for a second opinion. The doctor must make sure the patient has enough information to enable her to arrange to see another doctor. Best practice would include a letter to the next doctor. However, the GMC advice (in 2014) is that the doctor is not obliged to refer patients seeking abortion to other doctors who will authorise it – it's their opinion about the law, their conscience and your wellbeing that matters.[7]

- **Concerns about the doctor.** You have a right to a second medical opinion if you are not satisfied. When you see the doctor or nurse about a possible abortion and they seem rushed or unwilling to see you again to give time for reflection, you have a right to a second opinion.

- **Where information or advice is lacking** about potential physical, mental and emotional side-effects and the risks to near relationships or of provoking domestic violence; also information about the effects on fertility, your future children and your existing children – in writing. Ask yourself, 'Am I confident that this professional is expert enough to be making such a big decision on my health?' You are free to walk away.

- **If the law is not applied properly.** If you feel the law is not being applied as it should be, it is your right to ask for a second opinion. In best practice, you should be seen and assessed by two doctors before they sign the abortion form. As mentioned previously, recently information has come to light that some clinic doctors have been pre-signing forms without assessing women properly. This puts them and you at risk of being caught up in a legal case; but more importantly, it may put your health at risk.

Professionals with conscientious objection

A woman treated at an NHS hospital can expect to find around two thirds of the medical staff unwilling to be involved in abortions.[8] The hospital should have made provision for this before the woman is seen. The Abortion Act protects doctors who have a conscientious objection to involvement in abortion. But it does not stop a woman having an abortion if another opinion thinks she would be legal.

The Law in Northern Ireland, the Isle of Man and the Channel Islands

The Abortion Act does not extend to Northern Ireland, where most abortions are illegal except in limited cases where:

- It is necessary to preserve the life of the woman; or

- There is a risk of real and serious adverse effect on her physical or mental health, which is either long-term or permanent.

The Isle of Man and the Channel Islands have their own laws, distinct from the United Kingdom. In all these offshore islands, abortion has traditionally been largely prohibited, but this is under review.

Abortion Law in the USA, Canada and Australia

These three countries have abortion on demand in many of their states; globally this is rare. Nevertheless, as in the United Kingdom, the professionals must put the welfare of the woman first and supply all known information about the potential complications. Women have successfully sued their abortion doctor for 'failure to inform', in more than 20 cases in the United States and at least 3 cases in Australia.[9] And even if the risk is not generally accepted by the medical profession, legally, a physician must still present it to their patient as a potential risk. This is the legal doctrine of 'informed consent'.[10]

Abortion is legal up to and at birth in a few parts of the world such as Canada, some states in the USA and Australia – and in the UK in an emergency threatening the mother's life. Abortion providers are pressing for it in the UK. Abortion at birth is known as 'partial birth abortion', where the fetus is partly delivered like a birth through the vagina, before death. Then surgical destruction is done at that point to end the life of the fetus/child because the moment the baby is out that destruction would be legal murder.

The bottom line
Abortion law in England, Scotland, Northern Ireland and Wales – was designed to protect you, your unborn fetus and your existing family from a hasty decision and unsafe medical procedures. Since the English, Welsh and Scottish law is so ineffective, for your safety you must know your own after-effects of abortion.

But even in countries where there is legal abortion on demand, the duty of the health professional remains to provide informed choice, giving the couple or woman, in writing, information on *all* possible risks and complications, both short-term and long-term. Furthermore, professionals must not risk harm to any future children who may be put at risk by an abortion now of this their older sibling (see Chapters 12 'Overview of the After-effects of Abortion' and 21 'Premature Birth After Abortion).

Chapter 12
Overview of the After-effects of Abortion

This chapter covers:

- Physical health risks linked to abortion

- Mental, emotional and spiritual health risks

- Fertility issues after abortion

- Premature birth and other health risks for subsequent babies

In some situations, abortion may seem to be the only option, but before agreeing to one, you need to consider your future health. There is a whole range of after-effects – from immediate to lifelong complications. We looked at some of the immediate problems towards the end of Chapter 10 'Abortion Explored'; now we look in more detail at the longer term.

Please note carefully: the risks outlined here and further on in this book are *possible* after-effects. No one can say categorically that these things *will* happen to you; but some are more probable than others. It depends on many factors such as your age, previous pregnancies, existing health and STIs (sexually transmitted infections).

Miscarriage and abortion share some side effects, but there are many differences.

Science cannot say that abortion *causes* all these complications, but it can with some of them. Here we look at the major problems *linked* (associated) with abortion. It is quite a daunting list: if you have time to look into the more detailed chapters on each issue in Part 3 of this book, you may find they are not only connected to each other, but make sense. The chapters have tips on what you can do about some of the serious after-effects. For more detail, this overview chapter has pointers to other parts of the book.

All medical procedures carry some risk, as does pregnancy and giving birth, but evidence suggests that several side effects of abortion carry higher risk to your life and health than a full-term pregnancy and birth. Some of these raised risks may be long-term. Specialists have tried to add up all these risks to create an *overall raised risk* to life and health from abortion when compared to childbirth, but so far it has not been possible.

The elephant in the room

Any existing children, siblings of the fetus or stepchildren, will suffer loss from aborting the pregnancy. Evidence shows that in a family 'abortion is the elephant in the room'[1] which they long to talk about. Children can work out they would have had a sister or a brother who they will never know.'

The health risks linked to abortion can be broken down into four clusters:

1. Physical

2. Mental, emotional and spiritual

3. Threats to future fertility

4. Premature birth and other health risks for follow-on babies

Physical Health Risks Linked to Abortion
(For the early after-effects in the first few weeks after abortion, see Chapter 10 'Abortion Explored'.)

There has been much debate around the long-term risks of abortion, and the following come with evidence.[2]

- **Long-term pelvic pain** due to PID (Pelvic Inflammatory Disease) is linked to pain having sex. If you already have the Chlamydia infection, your likelihood of getting PID after abortion can rise to 7 women in 10. A study looking at nine previous studies showed that for women already carrying Chlamydia, those having legal abortion had the highest rate of going on to suffer from PID; this rate ranged from 27% to 72%.[3] Prior to abortion, Chlamydia screening should be done and should be treated with antibiotics if necessary. However, success of treatment is not guaranteed.

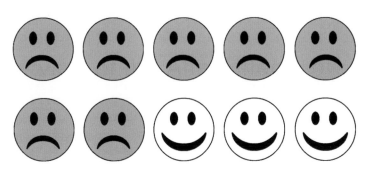

**Rate of possible PID after legal abortion
in 10 women with Chlamydia infection**

- **Breast cancer.** The question of whether abortion leads to a higher risk of breast cancer in later life is much debated. For this reason, Chapter 18 is devoted to the issue. In brief, research suggests that for a young woman who has never been pregnant, any issue, like abortion, which delays her first full-term pregnancy (FFTP) will bring a raised risk of breast cancer.

In a woman, every five years' delay in first full-term pregnancy is associated with an almost 20% increase in risk of breast cancer.[4] A well-known study in 2004[5] which said that there is no link between abortion and breast cancer has been overtaken by doubts. Since then 45 of 46 new studies up to 2016 have shown a positive link with abortion and breast cancer.[6] The claims of no connection by the Royal of Obstetricians and Gynaecologists College in 2011 were based on old research dating from before 2006.[7]

The 2001 Henriet study on French women who'd had more than one previous abortion showed their risk of cancer roughly doubles after the age of 34 years. This is due in part to being older first-time mums who are at higher risk. [8]

- **Failed abortion.** In some cases, the fetus survives the abortion attempts and may even be born alive. In 2008, 66 fetuses were born alive this way, and each year some survive to grow up.[9] (Read more in Chapter 16 'Physical After-effects of Abortion'.)

- **Perforation of the uterus.** This is when the surgeon accidentally makes a hole in the womb, and happens to between 1 and 4 women for every 1,000 abortions. However, worryingly this may be an underestimate.[10] The risk is lower when the surgeon is more experienced.[11]

- **Damaged lining of the womb** (Asherman's syndrome). This can happen after surgical scrapes (D and E) as part of the abortion procedure. A Chinese study found almost 4 women in 10 with Asherman's and infertility had had a previous abortion.[12] The concern is that it is linked to later miscarriages, adding to difficulties in producing a healthy baby when wanted.

- **Mortality rises among women after abortion:** Thankfully, death *during* abortion appears to be rare if there are high medical standards in use. But *after* abortion, the risks of early death over the next 10 years rises; and it rises more with each abortion. The average age of death for the women is 28. These are much higher risks to women's lives when compared to everyday risks like use of the roads. They are between 2 to 4 times higher than having a baby. (See more in Chapter 17 'Mortality of Women After Birth and Abortion'.)

More information on each of these issues can be found in Chapter 16 'Physical After-effects of Abortion'.

Mental, Emotional and Spiritual Health Risks

- **Major mental and emotional** health illnesses rise after abortion compared to after birth. Professor David Fergusson, who is known to be not opposed to abortion on conscience grounds, found there were small to moderate increases in risks of some major mental diseases like depression after abortion, even in those with no previous history of problems.[13],[14]

- **Suicide and self-harm** are more likely, and the father may be at higher risk of suicide as well.[15] See more in Chapter 19 'Mental and Emotional Effects of Pregnancy Loss'.

- **Regret and long-term guilt** can be experienced by both women and men, and this can continue even into their old age. It can be difficult to come to terms with such feelings, but in the right hands, help can be effective.[16]

- **Loneliness, isolation and economic hardship** may be eventual outcomes from the breakdown of close relationships following abortion.[17]

- **Guilt.** For those with a religious faith, guilt can affect domestic peace and ultimate wellbeing following abortion; resolving this can be difficult. If you are a Christian, abortion is not the 'unforgivable sin'. However, some Muslims believe it is. (Read more in Appendix 1 'ABC of Spiritual Beliefs on Pregnancy, Abortion and Healing'.)

One might ask whether the emotional and domestic strife following abortion is adding to the *raised mortality* in women in the years after? Evidence suggests that in the months after abortion and the next ten or more years, there are links to higher rates of suicide, accidents and murder. In addition, some 'natural causes' of death may be related – things like high blood pressure and stroke which may arise from stress and risk-taking behaviours. (See more in Chapter 17 'Mortality of Women After Birth and Abortion'.)

- **Domestic Violence** is complex and we only flag it here. A multi-country World Health Organisation study in 2005[18] and other studies showed that domestic violence is related to an increase in sexual risk-taking behaviour, adolescent pregnancy and induced abortion. Male partners may become aggressive – in some cases even murdering the woman. As early as 1997, Gissler and others found the link with murder after abortion was 4.33 (this is an odds ratio showing a strong connection) but following birth the connection was only 0.31.[19]

More details are given in Chapter 19 'Mental and Emotional Effects of Pregnancy Loss'.

Fertility Issues After Abortion

- **Inability to conceive again.** Evidence points to the risk of being unable to conceive again rising by about 7 times after abortion.[20] (See Chapter 20 'Infertility After Abortion' for more information.)

Premature Birth and Other Health Risks for Subsequent Babies

- **Damage to the cervix** (neck of the womb) can occur during the forced widening of the cervical channel for abortion. This can weaken the ability of the cervix to hold the fetus in the womb. The Royal College of Obstetricians and Gynaecologists puts the risk of damage at up to 1 in 100 surgical abortions.[21]

- **Miscarriages.** Cervical damage and retained products of conception may contribute to early miscarriages if conception occurs within 3 months of an induced abortion.[22] This would suggest it is better to delay conception longer than 3 months after an abortion. A 2014 study from China showed a raised risk of miscarriage of 156% for women who had had 2 or more repeat abortions. [23]

- **Infection of the womb and fallopian tubes.**[24] Following an abortion there is a greater risk of infection of the womb and fallopian tubes. This can block the tubes, which reduces the chances of conceiving again.

FALLOPIAN TUBE OBSTRUCTION

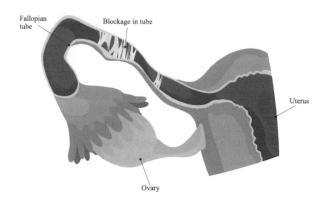

Fallopian tube   Blockage in tube

Uterus

Ovary

- **Ectopic pregnancies.** Ectopic pregnancy has been linked to previous abortion. Sadly, ectopic pregnancies cannot survive and must be removed to protect the woman's life. In 2006 an Australian study found that a woman's risk of ectopic pregnancy was 7–10 times higher after female infection and Pelvic Inflammatory Disease (PID), which are themselves linked to abortion.[25]

NORMAL PREGNANCY   ECTOPIC PREGNANCY

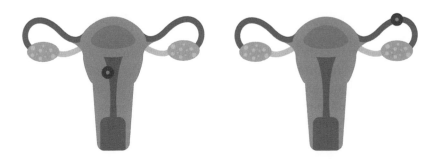

- **Stillbirth** of subsequent babies and life-threatening infections. Stillbirth is when the baby dies before or during birth. The link for abortion and these sad events may lie in the previous abortion procedure introducing infection, which lies quietly hidden till the next pregnancy. The risk of stillbirth increases by nearly 5 times after abortion, according to a Scandinavian study in 2003.[26]

- **The risk of placenta praevia** rises after one or more induced abortions. It means the baby must be delivered early to save the mother, so the baby may either not survive or be very premature, with all the problems that brings.[27]

- **Future preterm birth.** There is a risk to subsequent births from prior abortion, in that the surgical D&E (dilation and evacuation) of the womb, commonly done after abortion and miscarriage, has been linked to a two-thirds increase in risk of premature birth earlier than 32 weeks.[28] Babies that are born too early are at greater risk of cerebral palsy, infection and death. A study combining 37 other studies found that one previous abortion made a preterm birth in the follow-on pregnancy 27% more likely. Two or more previous abortions made preterm birth 62% more likely.[29] (See more in Chapter 21 'Premature Birth After Abortion'.)

Prevention is easier than cure

This chapter has given some bare statistics of problems linked to abortion that can be brought to life by countless stories online.

Meanwhile, other women and couples seem to go through abortion without apparent problem.

So, while both birth and abortion can bring either relief or challenges, you yourself need to weigh up in your own heart and head what is the right option for you, in the long term as well as the short term.

Chapter 13
Teenage Pregnancy and Abortion – Take Special Care

This chapter covers:

- Could you be pregnant?

- Which way forward?

- If you decide to have an abortion

- For parents and supporters of teenagers

- Young men

- Why are teenage abortion risks higher?

If you are a teenager, this chapter is for you

If you're reading this book on your own, you might find it helpful to get your mum, dad or a friend you trust to read it too, so that you can talk about it afterwards. Your body and feelings are still different from an adult in their 20s or older, so this chapter offers things to think over before deciding for abortion.

There is a section for parents in the second half of this chapter. As a parent, perhaps your daughter has just told you she is pregnant, or your son is now the father of an unborn child. Parents have hopes and dreams for their children – above all that they grow up into happy, confident adults.

Abortion in teens is linked with greater risks of physical and emotional problems than abortion in adults.[1] So, while abortion may be legally carried out on these vulnerable young women, handling this decision needs even greater care and caution.

In tragic situations like rape and abuse, it feels natural to do an abortion 'to remove the problem'. Sadly though, the clock cannot be turned back, the abuse cannot be undone, and all the abortion after-effects still apply. We must search for paths of care and healing that affirm the victim long-term and go to the roots of her distress.

A woman, pregnant as a result of rape, scoffed angrily at my offer to arrange abortion. Longer-term recovery is possible, as many women made mothers by or born after rape testify.

Could You Be Pregnant?

Are you a teenager and think you may be pregnant or your girlfriend could be? You may feel scared, especially about what your parents will say. Turn to Chapter 1 'Am I Pregnant?' for more information on how to find out whether you are pregnant.

If you are pregnant, you will feel shocked and numb for a few days. All kinds of thoughts and feelings will fly through your head. Keep calm, because with time and talking to trusted people there *is* a way forward.

Tell Mum and Dad if possible. Your parents and others should have your best at heart but they may not be aware of the medical side effects of abortion compared to having a baby. Teenage females' bodies are at special risk if they have an abortion, and you need to seek help before deciding. Side effects can be explored in other chapters of this book. (Look at Chapter 11 'Overview of the After-effects – Overview of Abortion.)

As a teenager, your vagina and womb are still growing and can be easily damaged by surgical instruments and drugs used in abortion. Germs can more easily get into your body than in older women. You are more vulnerable as a teenager to the serious side effects like bleeding, pain and emotional harm.

When you are a teenager, plans for having a family are probably way in the future, so you may feel hopeless and that your life is wrecked, finding yourself pregnant now. But contrary to what you might think, evidence suggests that having an abortion may worsen those feelings, while birth may improve them. Other issues also need to be weighed up, since having an abortion can make you more likely to give birth to a premature baby in the future, suffer from depression, and much later in life even breast cancer.

Which Way Forward?

Take time to think carefully about all your options. Going straight for abortion does happen, but will it solve your longer-term problems? Do you need it? Do you want it? Will it be safe?

Adoption of the baby, or temporary fostering after the baby is born, are alternative ways forward. And while your family may be shocked at first, they may rally round and say, 'We will help you look after this baby.'

Isabella's story

'I found I was pregnant in September, when I'd just turned 15, just before the school term started.

'I did the test in my bedroom. Everyone, all my family, was out. I just came downstairs and acted like I was fine.

'I went to school the next day and it really hit me then. I got really upset . . . the thought of it . . . I think I was quite numb for a while . . . it was very scary.

'I told my boyfriend, and that was it for a while . . . for about 2 weeks.

'We went to the health clinic and they were arranging an abortion straight away for me. They did not talk through any options but just gave me a leaflet and a follow-up appointment.

'My boyfriend was more scared than me, as his parents were stricter. I said I could not do it – have an abortion – and he supported me.

'As a teenage mum living at home, it's been hard to watch friends doing teen stuff and I feel I've missed out on those years. But I'm glad I kept my boy and now I know it's been the right thing.'

If You Decide to Have an Abortion . . .

For your own safety, it is best to let your mum and dad know. They can only help look after you properly if they know what's happening and what to look out for if you are suffering after-effects like felling upset, bleeding from below or get an infection, which can be serious.

Mum and Dad can let the clinic know about any family medical history or your own health history. The doctors at the clinic may not know enough information about your family to help you make a decision, and they probably don't have access to all your medical records. This story may help you see why:

Secret abortion

A junior doctor cared for a teenager who came into hospital for an abortion. She came with an older female friend and the parents were not to be told.

'Please don't tell Mum and Dad,' she said.

The doctor said, 'We will tell them it's a heavy period.'

After the abortion, she began to bleed heavily from her vagina. The consultant thought it might be retained parts in her womb and she went for another D and E . . . then another. Hormones were given to try to stop the bleeding. By now, the parents were visiting the hospital very concerned.

Each day the anxiety rose, and the web of lies to her family were becoming more and more difficult to sustain. Mum was asking, 'What is going on? Why can't she come home now?'

For Parents and Supporters of Teenagers

If you find your daughter is pregnant, keep calm! Talk it over with your partner, apart from your daughter at first, or if you are a single parent talk with a friend.[2]

Involve your daughter and the baby's father as soon as possible (the father has legal obligations until their child is 18). Nothing on earth can replace a parent's or friend's total, non-judgemental love and acceptance as your teenager works through the initial shock of pregnancy.

Legal criteria govern whether a teen aged under 16 can make her own decision about abortion. This may put your daughter at risk. In the UK, it comes down to whether she can understand the implications for both the short term and long term. Her own parents must be involved whenever possible. Winning the teen's trust and respect without pressure, storms or threats is an investment for life – theirs and yours.

New Zealand permits abortion for girls under 16 without parental consent. Even the pro-abortion Professor David Fergusson from New Zealand is unhappy with abortion 'on demand', without physician intervention, because he has uncovered the risks posed to mental health by abortion.[3]

Young Men
Some men are just as affected by abortion as some women. Numerous studies support this.[4] While some young men want nothing to do with it, others have a deep instinct to protect the girl and baby. As abortion goes against this, it can fuel deep shame, guilt and remorse,[5] so parents of the pregnant girl should try to involve his family if possible.

My teenage pregnancy – the pros and cons

'I had my son when I was 15, before I had even sat my GCSEs. The positives of having a child so early in my life are that he has kept me busy and given me the incentive to do better and get a good job. Being younger, I have had more energy to give and we shall be closer in age as we grow up.

'The negative aspects of teenage pregnancies are a lack of savings and difficulty in being able to afford things, along with the isolation from peers and loss of freedom which most teenagers enjoy.'[6]

Why Are Teenage Abortion Risks Higher?
The evidence shows that abortion in young girls is linked with greater risk of later emotional and physical problems compared to adults who undergo an abortion.[7] How do we know this?

Mental health and suicide – is birth or abortion safer?

Psychologist Patricia Coleman studied adolescent females' emotions. The youngsters showed less intellectual, moral and emotional maturity than adults. Events like a pregnancy are seen as having 'happened to' them rather than being the outcome of their own choices. When immaturity in thinking is coupled with limited ability to plan for the future, a teenager is more inclined to opt for an abortion.

However, a 2006 US study showed that adolescent girls who abort 'unwanted' pregnancies are five times more likely to seek help later on for psychological and emotional problems compared to their peers who carry 'unwanted' pregnancies to term.[8] And in high school students, suicide attempts were between 6 and 10 times more likely after abortion.[9] Teenagers are significantly less likely to attempt suicide *before an abortion* than adult women, but *after* abortion they are more than twice as likely as adult women to attempt it.

The following charts give you quick comparisons of how young women feel before and after a birth or an abortion. The slope of the line helps you grasp the change in their feelings from before to after.

Rate of attempted suicide per 1,000 young women:

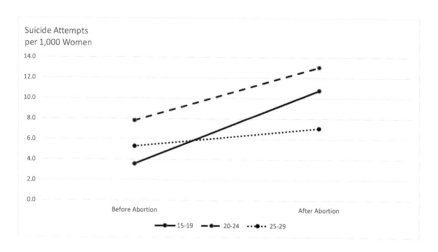

a) before and after abortion, by age group

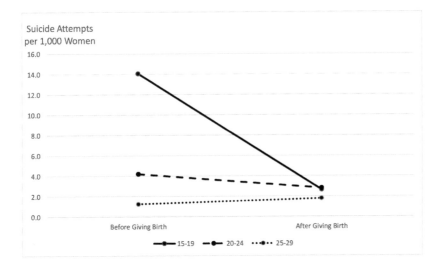

Suicide Attempts per 1,000 Women

15-19 ●—— 20-24 ●— 25-29 ··●··

b) before and after giving birth, for each of the three youngest age groups.[10]

Professor David Fergusson looked up the life outcomes for children until they were 25. He concluded, 'Abortion in young women may be associated with increased risk of mental health problems.'[11]

Important life decisions, such as having an abortion at a young age, can affect basic personality development – and may be connected with paranoia, drug misuse and psychosis later on.[12]

A nurse reports . . .

'I was doing routine summarising of notes for the family practice I worked for. I noticed a strong correlation between females who had major psychosis *in the year or two after* abortion, even though I was not looking for this finding and did not know of a link' (Sheffield, UK).[13]

Physical health after-effects of abortion

Way back in the 1980s it was known that teenagers were more likely after abortion to suffer infection of the womb, lacerations of the cervix and haemorrhage over half a litre of blood, compared to women aged 20 to 29.[14] Space permits only a small sample of other evidence.

When the STI chlamydia is present in girls aged 13–19 then a womb infection after abortion happens in over a quarter, compared to only a fifth of women in their twenties. Chlamydia is linked to later PID pain, infertility and ectopic pregnancy, and the fatality rates for ectopic are higher in women aged 15–19 than older women.[15]

In summary, in this chapter we have explored how teenagers are especially vulnerable in their bodies and as well as in their thinking. Abortion does not turn back the clock to get rid of the problem of unwanted pregnancy. Indeed there are serious health risks, and great caution is needed if considering abortion.

Chapter 14
Men, Pregnancy and Abortion

This chapter covers:

- Is what men think important in the pregnancy decision?

- What do men feel about pregnancy?

- What do men feel about abortion?

- Men's experience of abortion clinics?

- Will an abortion save a relationship?

- Where do men stand in law?

- Conflict between men and women

- Winners and losers?

Men? What has abortion got to do with men? Surely it's a women's issue, isn't it? . . .

This chapter explores how men feel about pregnancy and abortion and how men and women can cope well – or not – with the stress of an unplanned pregnancy dilemma and loss.

Jonathan Jeffes, founder of the Restore and Rebuild post-abortion course, has been counselling women and men about abortion for over 20 years. He reports, 'Generally, the experience of the women on our courses shows that a woman will nearly always go to the man involved, tell him she is pregnant and ask him what he thinks they should do as a couple. The reply often heard is: 'I will do whatever *you* want to do.'[1]

Is What Men Think Important in the Pregnancy Decision?

Jeffes' experience shows that underneath it all, abortion is about relationships. Since we have about 200,000 abortions a year in Britain, in many of these cases there are men involved in a close relationship with the women, even if briefly, and their thoughts and feelings about the pregnancy and a lifetime ahead should be considered.

Jeffes writes, 'Every journey begins with the first step. The journey to an abortion clinic does not just begin with the discovery of a pregnancy. It starts with a man and woman sleeping together, and it is here that men must also accept responsibility: for their behaviour towards women, in their values, in contraception and their understanding of abortion.

'These are not just 'women's issues', they are men's issues too, and whatever the story, men should be encouraged to face up to their part in an abortion decision.'

Does this help us understand why abortion can be an explosive issue between couples? Father's Day may not be easy for men after abortion.

> 'There is a myth in society that says men don't care. Or that men are untouched by the experience. My experience of having listened to men's stories over the years is that men are deeply touched by abortion loss but can't talk about it.' (A post-abortion counsellor)

In 2015, the programme *Long Lost Family* (ITV) showed a meeting at St Pancras Railway Station in London. The producers had brought together a French father and an English mother. The couple had last met one long hot summer, years before in France. The climax came when she gently confronted him, across the coffee table, regarding the abortion of their fetus that he had insisted on all those years ago. The confident, handsome man looked away; he looked at the floor; he struggled to speak, while guilt and sorrow swept over him.

In the same year, the *Times* newspaper reported on the new science of why dads matter: 'We now know that fathers' testosterone levels drop by up to 30% during their partner's pregnancies as they prepare to become caregivers; that fathers are more important than the mothers in children's language development . . .'[2]

So how do we understand the cause of anger that so often arises between men and women? Jeffes says, 'What is the difference between men and women?' He reports long discussions around this subject on his after-abortion courses but there is only one statement with which nearly everyone can agree:

> 'The men and women tell us that in a crisis a woman will look to a man for protection, and a man will instinctively want to protect her.'

This raises gender issues. But less encouragingly, he continues, 'Perhaps men also have an instinct to protect themselves from sacrificial responsibility. So, although initially a woman can think a man's response of 'Whatever you want' is supportive, later she may come to see this answer as a conscious withdrawing of the man's natural protection, and as a betrayal. She may also feel he is not protecting the child, as she instinctively wants to, even if she eventually chooses an abortion. This sense of betrayal is the powerful source of the anger that a woman can feel after an abortion.'

Unfortunately, it is often the case in dealing with pregnant women that the responsible male is nowhere to be seen. When I have been able to talk to the male partner of a pregnant woman seeking advice, and carefully explore their feelings, almost all were aware that they had a responsibility towards the woman and the fetus they had conceived between them.

What do Men Feel About Pregnancy?

Monica Heisy, in the British youth magazine *Vice*, said in 2014, 'In the few studies regarding the male reaction to the news of a pregnancy, their responses mirrored one of the most common responses of newly pregnant women: *ambivalence*. Ambivalence means unsure what to think and do now.

'Upon the discovery of a *hoped-for* pregnancy there is pride combined with fear, happiness combined with dread – both men and women tend to feel a mixture of angst and excitement.

'Confronted with an *unwanted* pregnancy these feelings, according to a Swedish study,[3] are almost the same as those reported by both men and women.'

'Men and women's reasons for *wanting to end a pregnancy* were also the same: wanting children later, wanting to be able to provide for their family at a level they felt comfortable with, being too young, or the more abstract, "It's not the right time".'

What do Men Feel About Abortion?

Monica Heisy tells of Paul, aged 28, who was at drama school when his girlfriend, a classmate, got pregnant . . .

'The experience was a bit like being painted out, unintentionally,' Paul told her.

Monica spoke to six men and discovered they all had a similar story to Paul's. They can often feel excluded from decisions regarding the pregnancy they have helped create.

Men's suicide has been observed directly after abortion, with a note linking the two events.[4]

Men's Experience of Abortion Clinics

Peter said, 'I had the kids with me, so they made me wait outside with them. I felt really upset as I wanted to support Alice. I took the view it was her decision, but I'm still haunted by it.'

Gary said, 'I went along with Jeanette to the abortion clinic. The whole place was run by women. They apologised but said they only had time for women.'[5]

In America, about 600,000 men go to the abortion clinic every year with their female partners. 'Men and Abortion' is an American website created to give men a voice on abortion. Research shows that about 6 in 10 men tend to be neutral but anxious before abortion. But afterwards some felt sad, lonely, guilty and powerless.[6]

Professor Arthur B. Shostak got interested after his own abortion clinic experience. He writes, 'Overall, the impact seems to have promoted ever greater protective ambivalence – a stressful mix of anxiety ('Will she be okay?'), puzzlement ('How did we ever get into this mess?'), and resolve ('I never want to be here again, never!').

'Here is the shock of finding oneself unexpectedly in a no-nonsense "no second act" drama, whereby the wellbeing of a loved one (in most cases) is actually in jeopardy, and the wellbeing of a barely glimpsed stranger (the fetus) is being resolved emphatically – almost regardless of whatever feelings the male may have toward his supposed offspring.

'The sense of powerlessness is great, and is aggravated by the loneliness of the men. Especially intriguing is the high percentage who report feeling guilty and sad.'[7]

The professor showed that men really wanted to talk about the whole business, especially afterwards. American clinics surveyed in 2005 had very few pamphlets available for men, yet men wanted counselling as well as the women. When the researchers questioned the clinics, they said that most of their staff were female and that they were not available to look after the men.

Will an Abortion Save a Relationship?
Couples often choose abortion in order to save their relationship, but will abortion deliver on that choice? A British counsellor said she knew several couples who are still together after abortion.

A psychotherapist answered the question this way: 'Unfortunately, all the evidence shows that abortion to "save a relationship" almost never works. Many relationships between couples come apart shortly after an abortion. These relationships often turn into prolonged, mutually destructive mourning rituals.'[8] Even married couples are often driven apart by an abortion, unless they can find a way to complete the grieving process together.[9]

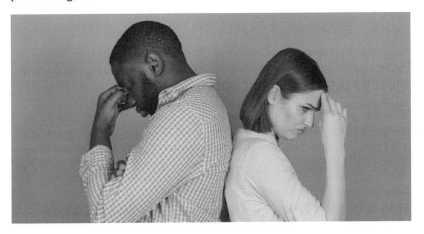

'Abortion breeds anger, resentment and bitterness toward the partner who was not supportive or who ignored their partner's desire to keep the baby.'[10]

Where do Men Stand in Law?
British law holds the man equally responsible with the woman for the child up to the age of 18. Yet, should the father want his unborn baby to be born and brought up, he has no authority in the law. The choice is made by others. Since he feels emasculated by the law, the easy way out is abortion, at which point he may leave and disappear from the scene.

Conflict Between Men and Women
Some men have used physical strength to abuse women because of a pregnancy that they have caused. Stories abound of women threatened into abortion or else . . . These powerful crosscurrents may break out in domestic violence – a huge issue which we look at in Chapter 19 'Mental and Emotional Effects of Pregnancy Loss'.

Winners and Losers?

- Couples working hard at their relationship before, during and after pregnancy can bring hope of a better long-term outcome.

- Although men don't feel the chemical and physical changes that a woman does in her pregnant body, they can feel deeply about the loss of abortion throughout their lives.

- Relationships in difficulty may be worsened by abortion.

- Fathers have no legal say in the abortion decision, so some can be left feeling helpless if a couple disagree over the decision.

- Abortion may seem the easier option, but afterwards the discord can divide partners and lead to loneliness and despair.

So who are the winners and losers after abortion on grounds of lifestyle choice? Estimates suggest some – perhaps many – men and women seem to feel relieved in the short term, and perhaps even in the longer term. For others, the human costs fall heavily on both sides of the relationship, and often their wider families.

You can find details of resources to help you get the support you need in Appendix 2 'Finding Help'. See also the website www.mendandabortion. com.

Chapter 15
Antenatal Screening and Disability in the Fetus

This chapter covers:

- Common screening tests and prenatal diagnostic tests

- Accuracy of diagnostic tests

- We parents decide on testing – don't we?

- What testing cannot do

- Abortion for fetal disability – does it help?

- Down's syndrome and similar conditions

- Finding help

This chapter is different because it covers dilemmas raised for parents where the child may be very much wanted, and questions raised by antenatal screening and potential disability. It looks at how you can work in partnership with professionals at the antenatal clinic, and the pros and cons of screening tests offered to all pregnant women.

Disability has become more accepted in the community in recent decades. It's quite understandable to dread the idea of giving birth to a baby with serious physical or mental disabilities, but for some time abortion has been used, in some cases, for problems that can be easily corrected, such as cleft palate or clubfoot. This, and the growing number of prenatal screening tests give parents-to-be a raft of dilemmas, not least, to test or not test? And would abortion be the best answer to the dilemmas or would it just add more difficulties?

One specialist said recently about testing, 'I have seen such benefit for parents, where they know they have a baby with an abnormality, happy to continue with the pregnancy but the knowledge has enabled best baby care and preparation of the parents.'

As soon as you go to tell your doctor or midwife you are pregnant, you will probably be faced with a question like, 'How do you feel about this pregnancy?' It's a way of getting you to think about whether you want an abortion or a baby. This chapter is about thinking that through before you meet it in the antenatal clinic.

Common Screening Tests and Prenatal Diagnostic Tests

Thankfully, most babies are 'normal'. The likelihood of a baby having a major problem such as Down's syndrome, spina bifida or heart problem is about 1 in 25.[1] Abortion for disability is accounts for about 1% of all British abortions – about 2000 fetuses a year. But perhaps worryingly, 'Clear evidence now shows that the main influence on the woman's decision to abort is the "attitude of the health professional giving the counselling after diagnosis".'[2] This chapter will help empower *you* to choose.

Fetal screening is offered for a range of conditions such as Down's syndrome, Edwards' syndrome and Patau's syndrome in the NHS programme. A blood test called the 'combined test' is offered at 10 to 14 weeks into the pregnancy. Cystic fibrosis testing is not routinely offered to pregnant women in the UK. Spina bifida and other physical problems are screened at the 'Fetal Anomaly Scan' at about 20 weeks into pregnancy. Spina bifida is a defect in the spinal column and it can range from very minor, causing almost no problems, to very major, with paralysis of the legs, bowels and waterworks. Women can take extra folic acid before and after conception to reduce the likelihood, as part of a healthy pregnancy diet (see more at https://www.nct.org.uk/pregnancy/pregnancy-nutrition).

While a mother may only want screening for reassurance that her baby is well, it is routine to discuss abortion if a problem is found. Ironically, the aim of helping parents-to-be happier and less pained (by means of abortion) may leave them suffering for years with less means of getting closure.

There's a difference between 'screening tests' and 'diagnostic tests'. Screening tests tell you the risk of your unborn having the problem screened for – either a numerical risk such as: 1 in 100 or description of risk such as 'high risk' or 'low risk'. But then your low risk might be your neighbour's high risk, depending how you feel.

A screening test cannot tell you that your unborn is *without* a problem, nor does it tell you the problem is *definitely* there. Despite the improvement in 'precision' technology, it is not uncommon for false alarms to be raised. I have seen or heard of several cases locally in recent years, and we meet one of these later in the chapter.

When the screening tests do raise some concern, then 'diagnostic tests' are usually offered to check the concerns about problems in the fetus. In most pregnancies, these tests are used at between weeks 11 and 25 of the pregnancy. In the much rarer, inherited diseases – the ones 'in the family' – such as Huntingdon's disease, they can be done quite early after conception, or even for studying the parents' genes before conception has occurred.

Diagnostic tests can put the life of the fetus at risk by provoking miscarriage. For example, in Chorionic Villus Sampling (CVS) commonly known as 'amniocentesis', the risk of losing the fetus is about 1 in 50 – and then the fetus may turn out to be healthy anyway.[3] It involves a needle being passed into the placenta for a sample, by going through the mother's tummy or through the vagina. CVS has several purposes, such as trying to confirm or exclude conditions like Down's or Edwards' – but it can be wrong either way.

Non-Invasive prenatal testing called NIPT
This is a screening test to look for problems in the genes. It is 'non-invasive' because it only needs a blood sample from a pregnant woman. Then they analyse the cell-free DNA (the genes) floating in the mother's blood. Direct 'invasion' of the unborn and the risk of miscarriage is avoided.

NIPT is not a sure diagnosis, nor is it a treatment. NIPT it is more accurate than other screening tests, but it can still be wrong. It's estimated that 1 in 10 pregnant women with a high chance of Down's syndrome will have false positive from NIPT, when the baby is normal.[4] This generates anxiety in the parents who may then decide to opt for the invasive test like CVS and risk miscarriage.

In the UK, women found to have a higher chance of Down's syndrome from the 'combined test' are offered NIPT at around 9 or 10 weeks' gestation. It can find about 97% of fetuses with Down's syndrome.[5] It can also show the sex of the baby and syndromes like Edwards', Patau's, cystic fibrosis and achondroplasia, where these are in the family.

Accuracy of Diagnostic Tests

The routine ultrasound scan offered to all pregnant women in the UK, the 'anomaly scan', is done at around 18 to 22 weeks. This test can be both a screening and a diagnostic test because it shows a high definition image of the baby.

The accuracy of ultrasound screening *correctly* detecting abnormalities 'incompatible with life' is 8 out of 10 attempts, while for 'serious abnormalities' where survival is possible 5 out of 10, and accuracy for those 'requiring immediate care' after birth it is only about 2 out of 10.[6]

Diagnostic tests for chromosome (gene) analysis are 98–100% certain. However, the uncertainty comes when 'mosaic' gene patterns occur. Mosaic genes are a mixture of good and bad genes, making it hard to predict what the baby will be like when born.

We Parents Decide on Testing – Don't We?

Protecting your freedom of choice in the face of these mysterious and powerful tests can be quite difficult. Some pregnant women and their partners refuse most screening tests. They say, 'Well we plan to care for this baby anyway, so we don't wish to have any screening tests which will raise doubts and dilemmas for us.'

If you choose the screening route, these are some of the questions to work through:

- Will this test make any difference to what we do in practice? You may say: 'We are going to look after this child whatever.'

- If there's a problem, would we choose abortion?

- If we were to choose abortion, how many aspects of the problem will that solve?

- Is abortion necessary for this problem? Will it cure anything?

- Are we trying to achieve the perfect child for others to see?

- Older women may feel they don't have so many chances left of pregnancy, healthy or not. How is that for you?

- Have we exhausted all possible treatments for the condition in the fetus?

- What is the *real* problem? Is it the inner disappointment I feel? Is it the effort or expense of long-term care?

- Having dug down to the real problems, be they financial, personal cost, sense of shame or disappointment – what options have we to solve those?

- Are we using a minor abnormality or a low risk of disease as a cover for some other reason? For instance, are we really feeling that this pregnancy is inconvenient?

- Will my partner and I, both now and later in life, feel that in a difficult situation we did the right thing and are content with that?

The research into screening is disturbing because it shows, unsurprisingly, that pregnancy has become a time of anxiety rather than joy. Several studies have shown that 8 out of 10 women were made anxious by screening.[7] The National Childbirth Trust (NCT) surveyed mothers' experiences of screening: 1 in 10 said they felt pressurised into having tests; they didn't feel that the test for disability in the unborn child was presented as a choice.[8]

So, while in the best centres choice is promoted, parents should find out all they can about these tests. Much more information is available online, for example at NHS choices and support groups for diseases.

A plan to go forward
To decide what testing you would like on your own pregnancy, think these questions over beforehand. Jot them down (perhaps at the back of this book) and then talk it over with the midwife or doctor, who will usually be only too happy to go along with your wishes. Think about how you feel, when some 'experts' may think that even the possibility of a disability puts 'the good mother under a duty to abort'.[9] Who is the expert – you or the

adviser who will not have to live with their choice? Most parents show an amazing desire to care for a disabled baby as best they can.

The positive side of screening

If, sadly, a serious problem is found before birth, then the parents can do some grieving and the healthcare team can prepare to cope. Usually specialists can supply written and verbal information to prepare people for the expected problem. Very occasionally, this involves actual treatment of the fetus before birth. In a fatal condition such as anencephaly, with major damage to the brain, delivery at the appropriate time can be arranged as part of planning terminal care for the baby, often in their mother's arms.

What Testing Cannot Do

Prenatal testing cannot always guarantee that the right diagnosis is made. And it cannot tell you how to make choices of the heart that it may present you with. That sort of guidance, applied with decision tools like the 4H in Part 1, comes from your heart beliefs on life and death, right and wrong, along with your cultural experience that make up your worldview.

Two doctors were expecting a baby. Annie and John (not their real names) heard at their 18-week scan that their baby showed a part missing from the brain. They were advised that abortion was the best option.

After much thought they decided, 'We are not sure these tests are correct – anyway we don't want to abort.'

Their baby underwent several more tests and the abnormality was downgraded to Down's syndrome. They waited . . . At 40 weeks, the mother delivered a girl. The baby doctor examined her carefully and announced, 'I think she is normal!'

She is now finishing primary school.

The best advice

A couple who were waiting for their results went to a counsellor. The counsellor said, 'Decide before the result what you will do.' As soon as they heard that it was clear: they knew they would keep the baby whatever the results and they would be well prepared for whatever was to come.

A correct diagnosis

Another couple were told that, sadly, their unborn girl had major disabilities and would live for only a few hours after birth.

They reluctantly decided to abort her early. They have since found the grieving prolonged and have complex feelings about the choice they made. Decades later, they still cannot easily discuss it.

Abortion for Fetal Disability – Does it Help?

Let's be aware of the pain and desperation in these choices. Abortion may bring a sense of relief, mixed with the sadness. Yet studies also show it brings a higher rate of depression in both mother and father; there is the guilt over what they have done added to the loss of self-esteem because they conceived an 'abnormal' baby. There is no reason to feel guilty about conceiving a disabled baby, nevertheless this sort of false guilt can be real.

Of course, there is terrible pain when a major disorder is found after birth. Having a disabled child can be devastating, and even break up a family. But it seems that the guilt and long-lasting after-effects for a number of women after any intentional ending of life can be even greater and longer lasting.[10] [11] The grief after these abortions can be as intense as for those women experiencing sudden loss of a child near birth.[12]

Down's Syndrome and Similar Conditions

Serious as the news is that you have a 'less-than-perfect' baby, the truth remains that every new life brings positives to our world. Down's syndrome is a useful example to illustrate this. Down's syndrome is one of the major abnormalities and caused by a problem in the genes, but many fears about it are based on wrong information. My friend was helping at a toddler's crèche and told me:

> 'Jimmy was the one with Down's syndrome. When Jimmy's mother came to collect him I said, "Jimmy has been happy and delightful to be with. But I'm afraid (smiling) two of the other toddlers have been howling non-stop whatever I do."
>
> "Oh, Jimmy is always easy," laughed the mum. "It's my other two that make me tear my hair out."'

Most people with Down's syndrome live into their sixties in fulfilled lives that contribute greatly to the community. Even so, most parents would prefer the struggles of a 'normal' child to those of a child with abnormalities. Like other inherited abnormalities, people with Down's syndrome come with a mixture of mental and physical disabilities that will mean a lifetime of special care. Online videos testify to the lives and careers that some of them are having. The *American Journal of Medical Genetics* reported research on children with disabilities and their families. They found that 99% of people with Down's syndrome are happy with their lives, more than three quarters of the parents had a more positive outlook on life, and almost 90% of the siblings said they consider themselves better people because of their family member with Down's.[13]

And don't we all need some care to survive through life? It's just a question of how much. I have visited adults with Down's syndrome in their middle years who are leading contented lives in caring communities.

Mohammed's Story

Mohammed and his wife have a little daughter Sara who is disabled with a condition like Down's syndrome. The couple are originally from a village in Pakistan.

'She is so special,' says Mohammed. 'When I put my shoes on to go out she says, "Da Da" and wants to come with me. She is without the jealousy of ordinary children, who say, "Hey, that's mine."

'She doesn't want to hurt anyone. All she needs is love. She gives to me something my other daughters don't give.'

With tears in his eyes he goes on, 'In my country I knew a family of microcephalics. We treated them as special people. They had something that others don't have. They were content with just food and water, far more content than everyone else.'

Writing this chapter as a doctor has reminded me of stories that have astonished and moved me. I remember parents-to-be coping with long anxious weeks with great courage – weeks that turned to years. My cousin

Peter's wife Brigid gave birth to Benjamin. Totally disabled, he was given four years to live. When he died in his twenties, after receiving devoted care all his life, his funeral was packed with tearful people who had seen and found significance in him and from him.

Finding Help

Parents-to-be who have these tests and face an unexpected problem need much support. This burden cannot be carried alone. A life-affirming environment will help – a place where their child will be welcomed and supported with loving care and acceptance. Churches, families and other social and religious groups can provide this long-term in ways the state can ever match.

Almost every problem that can arise in the unborn child has a website to provide help and support, and can be found online by a simple search.

Part 3
Informing Choice by Digging Deeper

Chapter 16
Physical After-effects of Abortion

This chapter covers:

- Cause and effect?

- Pain following abortion

- Painful sex longer-term

- Risk of serious infection after abortion or birth

- Pelvic Inflammatory Disease (PID)

- Reproductive organs: risk of damage

- Failed abortion and fetus survival

In this chapter we will start by looking at the short-term (that's in the first few weeks) physical after-effects mentioned in Chapter 10 'Abortion Explored'. Then we will look in more detail at the longer-term after-effects that were outlined in Chapter 12 'Overview of the After-effects of Abortion'.

Women may come through abortion just fine. Everyone is an individual and reacts differently. To keep this perspective, take infection as an example. It may help to remember that if you take 100 women, the risk of getting an infection will be about 10 women in those hundred. However, the *consequences* for the 10 with infection can range from mild discomfort to serious, including threats to fertility, even life-threatening.

All medical procedures carry risk, as does pregnancy and giving birth.

As we saw earlier, medical abortion has been reported to have 4 times more adverse after-effects in the 6 weeks after abortion than after surgical abortion.[1] Research has shown that 20% of women had some sort of adverse effect in the first 6 weeks after medical abortion. This is well above the claims of abortion providers such as the RCOG. And that was not counting *pain* for the woman, which is reported by between 25% and 50% women after abortion.[2]

Cause and Effect?

In most case, we can only point out *links* between abortion and specific health complications. In a few, we can say that some leading experts see true *cause and effect* – for example, breast cancer and preterm birth after abortion. In these cases, it is because experts have crunched the numbers and fulfilled the scientific conditions needed to prove that there is a connection.

Pain Following Abortion

Pain is a natural signal that something needs attention. It is common during healing. No one can say the exact level of pain you will feel after an abortion, but there will be some, and it may be severe. The reason is that both medical and surgical abortion involve stretching open the tightly closed neck of the womb, which is naturally contracting to keep the fetus inside.

In an Aberdeen study, 1 in 4 British women who'd had an abortion rated the pain 'as bad as it can be'.[3] In the USA, one in 2 women having a medical abortion reported the abdominal pain to be 'severe'.[4]

The number of American women reporting pain to be severe during medical abortion

> **RED FLAG**
>
> **Pain**
>
> Persistent or severe pain may be warning you of a serious side effect like internal bleeding or a punctured organ. Don't endure it alone or at home – see your doctor the same day.

Other reasons affecting the level of pain. Women can suffer with increased pain at abortion if they are anxious, or if it has been a long procedure. Even the atmosphere in the clinic can worsen pain.[5] Research shows that pain following abortion is more likely for younger females, those for whom it is their first pregnancy and those of white race.[6] Women having an abortion under sedation (drug-induced drowsiness) seem to suffer more from stress disorder, depression and physical ill-health 1 month after abortion and 3 months afterwards than those having a general anaesthetic (fully unconscious).[7]

Painful Sex Longer-Term

Abortion, as with other gynaecological procedures, brings the risk of germs getting in. In the short-term, sex can be too painful to attempt if infection in your pelvic organs gets a grip. These germs can cause Pelvic Inflammatory Disease (PID), which is marked by longer-term pain and repeated vaginal discharge. If there is Chlamydia there, the rate of PID after abortion can rise to 7 women in 10.[8] PID is linked to experiencing painful lovemaking for the woman.

Risk of Serious Infection After Abortion or Birth

In March 2017, the Health Secretary for the UK government, Jeremy Hunt, announced:

> **RED FLAG**
>
> **Infection**
>
> 'Every death from sepsis (life-threatening infection) is a tragedy, yet too often the warning signs are missed.' Secretary of State for health, 2017

Even with the best care in the world, infection can get a grip, which is why the Secretary of State for health sent the above message to the NHS and the people of Britain. So, if you have just had an abortion or a baby and you feel weak, clammy, over hot, feverish or cold call your doctor. Treatment should be started within the hour.[9]

Pelvic Inflammatory Disease (PID)

PID can scar the fallopian tubes and so block future conception, making the woman infertile. Another problem is that whilst these blocked tubes might allow conception, the embryo cannot move down into the womb, causing an 'ectopic pregnancy', which is dangerous and one of the commonest causes of death in women who are pregnant.

Overall, in 100 women with PID, 18 will suffer chronic pelvic pain, 12 will suffer infertility and 8 will have an ectopic pregnancy.[10]

So, you should tell your personal doctor immediately if you any fever, vaginal discharge or abdominal pain (tummy ache) after an abortion.

Reproductive Organs: Risk of Damage

As we have seen, surgical abortion can tear the neck of the womb and puncture the womb itself or the bowels around the womb. This sort of damage is a threat to the woman's wellbeing and fertility.

In a study of 6,408 abortions, US researchers found that puncture of the womb had occurred seven times more often than the abortion surgeons had thought.[11] Punctures can lead to infection around the bowels and serious peritonitis. Peritonitis can leave the organs in the pelvis painfully stuck together, this is known as 'adhesions'. Adhesions can contribute to pain during sex and fertility problems long after abortion.

Failed Abortion and Fetus Survival

'Failed abortion' commonly means parts of the fetus are left behind in the womb with the risk of infection and bleeding. Further surgery by D and E is needed.

Much more rarely, the fetus survives the abortion attempt and is born alive. In 2008, 66 fetuses were born alive this way, and each year some survive to grow up. This figure for babies born alive after abortion came from the UK government's Confidential Enquiry into Maternal and Child Health.

Chapter 17
Mortality of Women After Birth and Abortion

This chapter covers:

- Women's mortality during the 10 years after birth or abortion

- Where the evidence comes from

- Comparing life scenarios for risks from abortion and birth

- Why might abortion be linked to death?

Evidence from many studies suggests that women have higher rates of dying in the 10 years after abortion compared to the 10 years after giving birth. Risks are raised by miscarriage as well, but less so than abortion.

Thankfully, death *during* the abortion procedure appears to be rare where there are high medical standards being practiced.

Women's Mortality During the 10 Years After Birth or Abortion

First look at this bar graph to compare the number of women's deaths in the 10 years after birth compared with women who had abortions. Women in their first pregnancy, who ended it with an early or late abortion had significantly higher mortality rates over the next 10 years.[1]

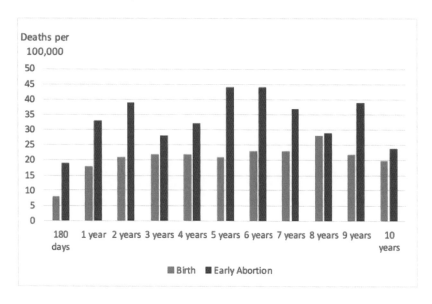

Death rates following first pregnancy outcome at 180 days and during each of first through tenth years after pregnancy outcome[2]

Women who give birth are less likely to die than those who don't become pregnant, those who have had an abortion and those who have miscarried.[3]

Another study carried out among low-income women in California confirms this mortality risk. It looked at 8 years of a woman's life after abortion compared to birth. The mortality rate for women who had a live birth after a previous abortion was 462 per 100,000, while for women who had abortions during the same time frame, it was 854 deaths per 100,000, or about double the risk.[4]

More encouraging, this study of women in California and another in Denmark (over a million women)[5] suggests that giving birth after previously having an abortion may help reduce the higher risk of dying connected to previous abortions and miscarriages.

Where the Evidence Comes From
Denmark and Finland have excellent medical records. There, a woman's whole life can be followed up to death and can be linked with her pregnancy history, including abortion and her death. Great Britain and the

USA are not equipped for such studies due to deficient medical records. For instance, in the British NHS, the woman's NHS number cannot be easily linked with her history of abortion, so abortion mortality cannot be properly studied – requests to instate this simple measure have been rebuffed so far.

Comparing Life Scenarios for Risks from Abortion and Birth

Abortions later on in pregnancy are riskier than early abortions

There is consensus that abortions carried out late in pregnancy are linked with a) more short-term after-effects on the woman's health (see chapter Abortion Explored) and b) higher rates of death compared to early abortions.[6]

Pregnancy losses raise women's mortality in the first year after the loss

Death rates were higher in women who had any loss, either from miscarriage or abortion, than the non-pregnant or those who had a birth at full-term pregnancy.[7],[8]

Let's compare that with the risk of road death in the UK in one year to September 2014:

- The risk of dying on a UK road in the year 2014 was 2.9 in 100,000.[9]

- The risk of dying in a single year after an abortion was found to be 82 in 100,000.

This figure was published in 2004 from Finland after adjusting for the woman's age.[10]

Now, if you look at a typical 'risk statement', such as the ones provided in pill packets, a risk of less than 1,000 bad outcomes per 100,000 people is described as an 'uncommon' risk. But when an 'uncommon' occurrence is as severe as death, it is an important risk for the women and their families who are the unlucky victims.

These deaths after abortion seem mostly to be happening as a result of self-destructive or risk-taking behaviours (which women may not be aware of at the time). But if they had all given birth, the evidence suggests a lot more of them would still be alive 10 years later.

Repeat abortions compared to repeat births

The following charts compare the relative long-term mortality of women after a) births and b) abortions.

Women's Long-Term Death Rate

(adjusted for year of woman's birth, age at last pregnancy and number of exposures to each of the other pregnancy outcomes)[11]

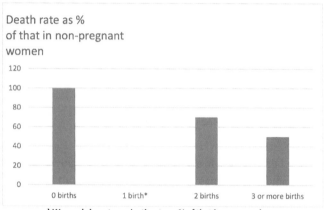

a) Women's long-term death rate as % of that in women who are not pregnant ('0 births'), for women with different numbers of births
* Not available from source

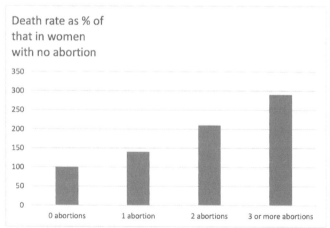

b) Women's long-term death rate as % of that in women who have had no abortions, for women with various numbers of abortions

Women's long-term death rate
(adjusted for year of woman's birth, age at last pregnancy and number of exposures to each of the other pregnancy outcomes)
Source: Table 3 of Coleman PK, Reardon DC, Calhoun BC. Reproductive history patterns and long-term mortality rates: a Danish, population-based record linkage study. *Eur J Public Health*. 2013;23(4):569-574. doi:10.1093/eurpub/cks107.

NB: these two bar charts have different scales on the left hand vertical column. The death rate, for comparison purposes, is given a figure of 1.0. So the bar heights give you an 'at a glance' comparison with women who had 0 to 3 births (top chart) and women who had 0 to 3 or more abortions (lower chart). There is no bar for the women having 1 birth because there was not enough data to use.

You can see that repeat abortions bring extra risks whereas repeat births tend to bring extra benefits by lowering the mortality risk.

Abortion or birth – what are the risks during the next 25 years?

A Danish study in 2012, on over 1 million women,[12] followed the mortality rate for 25 years after the end of pregnancy. There were statistical controls for the number of pregnancies, birth year and age at last pregnancy. They showed that:

- One abortion brought a moderate raised risk of dying, at 45% higher. This risk to the women was detected from 180 days after the loss and onwards.

- One natural miscarriage also brought moderate raised risk of dying but less than from abortion.

- More than one abortion showed a moderately high increased risk of early death (average age 28) compared with no abortion. But 2 abortions brought *double* the risk of no abortion and 3 abortions brought about *triple* the risk.

- Women who gave birth to 2 and 3 or more babies, had about half the death rate of those not pregnant.

Why Might Abortion be Linked to Death?

It's realistic to ask why abortion, and to a lesser extent miscarriage, could be linked to deaths in young women after the event? Remember, these studies counted the deaths from *all causes*. The risks were mainly from 'outside' causes such as suicide, murder and accident, rather than causes like bleeding or infection from the abortion inside the woman's body.[13,14,15]

But some died of 'natural' causes – things like high blood pressure and strokes. Perhaps these may be stress-related from the loss of the fetus.[16,17]

More information on *suicide* after pregnancy loss can be found in Chapter 19 'Mental and Emotional Effects of Pregnancy Loss' and Chapter 13 'Teenage Pregnancy and Abortion – Take Special Care.)

In conclusion

All these studies show that we cannot be complacent about risks to the actual life of the woman in the years after abortion. These are high when compared to risks from everyday life such as road accidents. And the risks are 2 to 4 times higher than having a baby.

Chapter 18
Abortion and Breast Cancer – Is There a Link?

This chapter covers:

- Abortion and breast cancer – the key factor

- The age of first full-term pregnancy (FFTP) factor

- Other lifestyle factors fuelling the rise in breast cancer

- Why is abortion and breast cancer connected?

What you need to know

In England, female breast cancer is the commonest cancer in women and rising. In 2015, there were 45,000 new cases of malignant cancer – that's about London's Wembley stadium half-full. These happen most often in women between the ages of 15 and 60 years.[1] Thankfully, about 85% of those who do get it are expected to survive for at least 5 years with expert care.[2] The risk of a woman getting malignant breast cancer at some time during her life was about 1 in 8, but by 2017 this had risen to about 1 in 7 women.[3] If one counts women with pre-cancer changes this is now close to 1 in 6 women.

Abortion and Breast Cancer – The Key Factor

For any woman considering abortion, the *key factor* is the age at which she has her first full-term pregnancy (FFTP) – the older she is, the more likely she is to suffer breast *cancer*. So, delaying having a baby, for example by having an abortion earlier on in life, is increasing her age for that FFTP and therefore increasing her chances of getting breast cancer, as 3 studies show.[4]

The women most affected by this breast-cancer concern are those in their teens, twenties and early thirties, especially if they are pregnant for the first time. And also those who may be older, but had an abortion in their teens, twenties or early thirties, and especially if it delayed a first full term pregnancy. That's because the risk persists for life.

The idea of the abortion–breast cancer (ABC) link surprised me, because here specialists are saying that abortion *causes* the cancer rather than there being a loose association or link.[5]

British specialists have until now been reassuring people that there is no link, but this is usually based on a study from 2004.[6] In the 10 years of research from 2006 to 2016 there were 46 peer-reviewed scientific studies involving the abortion–breast cancer link. All, except one, found that previous abortions raise the breast cancer risk (these studies are listed on our website http://www.choicescommunity.com).

Repeat abortions raise cancer risk

Evidence also suggests that the more abortions a woman has, the greater the risk of breast cancer. It's like smoking. We know smoking raises the risk of lung cancer and the more you smoke the more likely you are to get lung cancer. Abortion also shows this 'dose effect' on a woman's risk of breast cancer: the more abortions a woman has, the higher the risk of breast cancer cells growing.

A Chinese study in 2012 showed the 'dose response' phenomenon, with 2 abortions being riskier than one. They found that women who had had a previous abortion experienced a 33% increase risk for one abortion, 76% for two abortions and 165% for three or more abortions.[7]

In 2017 headlines announced, 'British breast cancer epidemic correlates with fertility and induced abortion . . .' in the *Journal of American Physicians and Surgeons*.[8]

Huang's study of 46 studies in 2014 concluded that one abortion increases the woman's risk of breast cancer by as much as 44%.[9]

The Age of First Full-Term Pregnancy (FFTP) factor

The increased breast cancer risk in women who never get pregnant has been known about since the seventeenth century. Modern studies on this age of first full-term pregnancy factor have been accepted, for more than 25 years. For instance, back in 1983 the study by Trichopolous of about 17,000 women, showed that in a woman every five years' delay in full-term pregnancy is associated with nearly one-fifth increase in risk of breast cancer.[10]

> Each 5-year delay in FFTP adds one-fifth greater risk of breast cancer.

The authors say, 'There is evidence that the age of approximately 35 years represents for every birth a critical point; before this age any full-term pregnancy confers some degree of protection; after this age, any full-term pregnancy appears to be associated with increase in breast cancer risk.'[11]

It is not just because she is older, and not because she is not breastfeeding, although having a baby early in life and breastfeeding are known to protect against breast cancer.

Take Alice for example:

Imagine a young woman called Alice. Let's suppose she gets pregnant for the first time in her life aged 25 but ends it with an abortion at 12 weeks. If she waits five years to give birth to her first baby at the age of 30, then she is *20% more likely* to get breast cancer later in life than if she had carried the first pregnancy to full term. If she waits ten years, till she's 35, then she is *40% more likely* to get breast cancer.

> Doubling the woman's age delay from five years to ten years later for her FFTP, roughly doubles her increase in breast cancer risk over her lifetime.[12]

But could it simply be that Alice's breast cancer risk is just higher because she is older when her first baby is born? After all, the longer she lives, the more time available to draw the short straw for cancer.

No, this is probably not the case. There are 3 or 4 *independent* risk factors explaining why delay in FFTP can be linked to higher risk of breast cancer:

1. Alice is older when she has her first full-term pregnancy, which delays the potential breastfeeding protection.[13]

2. Alice is interrupting her pregnancy in the first trimester (first 12 weeks).

3. Alice has a higher risk of premature birth (born before 32 weeks' gestation) in any follow-on pregnancy, and this is in itself an independent risk for breast cancer. This was shown by Melbye who is well known in this field.[14]

What about Alice's breast cancer risk if she has a miscarriage?

If she loses the baby through miscarriage in the first 12 weeks, then she *does not suffer such a large rise* in risk of later breast cancer as having an abortion. (However, miscarriage in the middle trimester of pregnancy does carry a higher risk of later breast cancer.) The explanation is probably to do with hormones. Early miscarriages are often in women with low oestrogen hormone so the breasts are not made prone to cancer by the oestrogen.

Other Lifestyle Factors Fuelling the Rise in Breast Cancer

A woman's hormones seem to be the most important cause of cancer change in women's breasts. That's why abortion *and* the following factors can increase your risk:

- The older you are at the time of your FFTP.

- Starting your periods early in life is a factor increasing breast cancer risk.

- Breastfeeding a baby is protective against breast cancer and the longer the better, but lower fertility in recent years means fewer women breastfeeding.

- Hormone replacement therapy (HRT) and the oral contraceptive pill both bring a similar higher relative risk of breast cancer. A woman's risk doubles with either of these, so that by the age of 50, her risk of breast cancer rises to 1 in 25 women not 1 in 50.[15] The lifetime risk is much higher again, at 1 in 6 or 1 in 7, as we saw at the start of the chapter.

- Family history matters. About 5–10% of women inherit a gene that is linked to breast cancer which needs specialist genetic advice.

Why is the abortion–breast cancer link not better known?

Leaving aside commercial interests, doctors are still much influenced by Professor Valerie Beral's study back in 2004.[16] However, errors in her methods have been publicised (including in the British Parliament in 2007[17]). Firstly, Beral's team overlooked the fact that women can lower their breast cancer risk by breastfeeding[18] – if women have an abortion, the protective period of breastfeeding is lost.

Secondly, they overlooked the accepted research that the older the woman is at FFTP, the higher her risk of breast cancer.

Thirdly, Beral was quoted as saying, 'Scientifically this is a full analysis of the current data.'[19] Yet important studies were left out and unchecked studies put in.[20]

Why is Abortion and Breast Cancer Connected?

Back in the seventeenth century, it was noticed that Italian nuns who had never been pregnant were more likely to get breast cancer.[21] We now know that one reason for this is the protection to the woman that comes from carrying a pregnancy to full term. This is because a sequence of changes happens in the breasts when a woman goes through a pregnancy, to get ready to provide milk for a baby. The breast creates more tissue ready to do this, which is why breasts get bigger during pregnancy. This new breast tissue is vulnerable to cancer – but only for a time – because it can be reversed to a safer state than before. This reversal is achieved by the older fetus and placenta.

So, a young woman who has never been pregnant (like those Italian nuns) has breasts which are already more prone to develop a cancer. Early pregnancy then makes the breasts even more cancer-prone. But, if the pregnancy goes beyond 32 weeks then her breasts change from 'cancer-prone' to 'cancer-resistant'. There is a critical amount of time to achieve this change and it is those first 32 weeks of pregnancy. So long as she gets *beyond 32* weeks, the cancer-prone breast tissue has a chance to mature into cancer-resistant. This is because around this time the older fetus and placenta produce a hormone called 'human placental lactogen' (HPL), which helps breast cells become cancer-resistant.

Any pregnancy that ends before 32 weeks, through any means, stops this tissue change from completing; the woman is left with breast tissue that has become even more at risk of becoming cancerous than if she had never been pregnant at all. These cells remain cancer vulnerable for the rest of her life. Abortion cannot remove these cells.[22]

If the woman breastfeeds her baby, then her cancer protection is increased even more than the protection of having a full-term birth.[23]

Why pregnancy changes the breast tissue. During pregnancy, hormones such as oestrogen, which stimulates breast cancer cells, have been released around the body in larger quantities than before the pregnancy. The NHS website states, 'Your risk of developing breast cancer may rise slightly with the amount of oestrogen (estrogen) your body is exposed to.'[24]

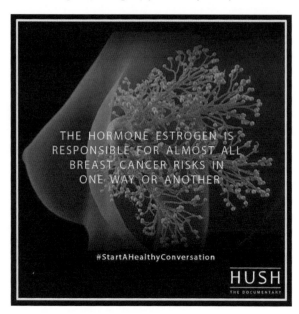

THE HORMONE ESTROGEN IS RESPONSIBLE FOR ALMOST ALL BREAST CANCER RISKS IN ONE WAY OR ANOTHER

#StartAHealthyConversation

HUSH
THE DOCUMENTARY

Healthy Irish women have fewer breast cancers

This benefit from fewer abortions may benefit nations. In 2007, the *Journal of American Physicians and Surgeons* showed that abortion was the greatest predictor of breast cancer frequency in nine European countries: England, Wales, Scotland, Northern Ireland, the Irish Republic, Sweden, the Czech Republic, Finland and Denmark.[25]

Irish women, have been shown to have lower risks of breast cancer, at 1 woman in 10 before the age of 75,[26] than women in England and Wales[27] – until recently, few Irish women had abortions. Studying the breast cancer epidemic, British statistician Patrick Carroll found that since 1968, when abortion numbers in England and Wales soared, English and Welsh women suffered a parallel increase (but delayed by some years) in breast cancer rates,[28],[29] while there was a much lower rise in rates of breast cancer in Irish women. Remember, there will be a delay before the increase in abortions shows up in cancer rates, because cancer is delayed some years after the abortion.[30]

Breast Cancer Epidemic

'The link is very close between rates of abortion and rates of breast cancer in all the countries with good health records of abortion and cancer. This is evidence.'[31],[32]

Dr Patrick Carroll, Statistician

On the other hand, the more full-term pregnancies a woman has, the more protected she is from developing breast cancer. A Swedish study in 1996 showed that each baby born lowers a woman's risk of breast cancer by another 10%.[33]

Self-help tips to catch cancer early[34]

Regular self-examination may help find and treat any breast cancer early. If you've had an abortion, or a first full-term birth later in life, then it's even more important. In Britain, all women get called for screening after the age of 50 and it is important to attend.

Get to know how your breasts normally feel and look so you will be more likely to spot any changes that could be signs of breast cancer. When you check your breasts, also feel for swellings or lumps in the armpit.

The top three symptoms you should report early are:[35]

- Feeling a lump in your breast: 90% of cancers are found this way.

- A painful lump in the breast: 20% of cancers are painful.

- Nipple change or discharge: 10% of cancers have this symptom and some have a skin change around the nipple that looks like eczema. The nipple might be pulled back into the breast, or change shape, you might have a rash that makes the nipple look red and scaly.

Black-American women are more likely to get an aggressive form of breast cancer termed 'Triple Negative Breast Cancer' (TNBC) than Caucasian women.

> A 2017 study found that Black-American women who breastfeed over 11 months cut their TNBC odds by nearly half.[36]

Other factors you may have some control over to lower your risk of breast cancer:

- Regular screening is available on the NHS after the age of 50.

- Breastfeeding is a protector against breast cancer, and so abortion would remove the breastfeeding protection.

- Sadly, premature birth itself is a risk factor for breast cancer.[37] Premature birth (birth before the fetus is 32 weeks' old) – which is more common after previous abortion – leaves the breast tissue in a cancer-prone state.

- The use of hormone contraceptive pills and HRT (hormone replacement therapy) increase a woman's risk of breast cancer.

Regular breast screening by mammogram can catch cancer early.

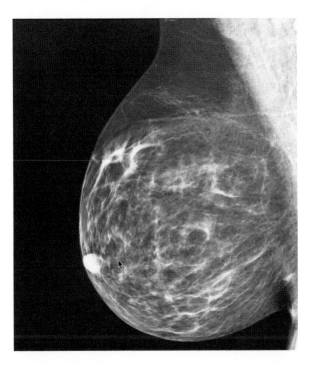

In 2011, the Royal College of Obstetricians and Gynaecologists (RCOG), when they were taking advice on what to say in their evidence-based clinical guideline 'The Care of Women Requesting Induced Abortion', were told by one of their peer reviewers, Professor Joel Brind PhD: 'Women should be informed that induced abortion leaves women – especially childless women – at significantly greater risk of future breast cancer, compared to carrying the pregnancy to term.'

In conclusion

Abortion is not the only factor in the rise of breast cancer in the last 50 years, but there is growing evidence of a link with breast cancer. And not only a link but cause and effect. In the 35 statistically significant studies up to 2013, one sees the nine Bradford Hill criteria for causation fulfilled. When these strict criteria are met we can conclude that abortion is a *cause* of breast cancer, not just linked with it or positively associated with it. Sir Austin Bradford Hill established these criteria in 1964 and used them to show that lung cancer was caused by cigarettes. [38]

Chapter 19
Mental and Emotional Effects of Pregnancy Loss

This chapter covers:

- Mental Health

- Recent news on mental health risks

- Red flag mental health warnings before choosing abortion

- Suicide and Pregnancy Loss

- Close relationship breakdown after abortion

- Mortality concerns after abortion

Introduction
This purpose of this chapter is to help you weigh up your own risks of mental and emotional ill-health that might come after an abortion compared to after having a baby. Emotions are a complicated part of life and saying birth or abortion *caused* depression, or relief, is often not so clear.

Most people admit that abortion is unpleasant to go through. While many women feel short-term relief after the abortion, a greater concern might be your longer-term mental health and peace of mind. People experiencing abortion for severely abnormal babies are just as at risk as those seeking 'social abortion' – in fact may be more at risk (see Chapter 15 'Antenatal Screening and Disability in the Fetus'). Talking over your feelings with someone before deciding whether to have an abortion can help you make your choice, as we explored in Part 1.

> ## RED FLAG
>
> ### Mental Health Warnings Before Abortion
>
> Past or present mental health problems in a woman are a Red Flag of caution if she is considering abortion. If a woman has had mental health problems before abortion she is more likely to have major mental health problems afterwards.

Mental Health

In the UK 99.5% of abortions are performed under the legal requirement that it will *improve* your mental health, but this is hard to prove one way or the other. Without doubt, some factors raise the risk of *damaging* rather than improving mental health following the abortion.[1] There is a checklist later on in this chapter.

Range of emotions

Most family doctors have seen women showing a range of emotions after abortion, from relief, to mild tearfulness, to extreme grief up to decades later. Counsellors have called it a loss that is difficult to acknowledge, 'a disenfranchised grief' because it's a choice the woman has made herself. This makes it difficult to talk about, because there's the belief that all is okay now that the abortion is done – or it should be.

Recent News on Mental Health Risks

A major British review into mental health after abortion in 2011, based on thorough research, found that having an 'unwanted' pregnancy is linked with increased risk of mental health problems. If the woman then goes on to have an abortion, this raised risk of mental health problem is *still there*, as it would be if she had given birth.[2] So all women with an unwanted pregnancy need support and care, and it would be wrong to assume that abortion will solve a mental health problem related to that situation.

These cautions were backed up by New Zealand Professor David Fergusson in 2013, who re-examined the British review. Fergusson is known to favour abortion without conscience grounds. He and others found there were small to moderate increases in the risk of some mental health problems post-abortion, even in women with *no previous history of problems*.[3],[4]

These problems include major depression, suicidal tendency and substance misuse. Back in 2008 he spoke of a small 'causal' link between abortion and mental ill-health after a 30-year follow-up study on women.[5] He says abortion does not improve mental health.[6] He advocates that the law should insist on a physician advising women of the risk to their mental health before abortion.

Post-abortion counsellors sometimes see women with previous mental stability experiencing deep distress. In contrast, no other pregnancy results, such as miscarriage or having a baby, were consistently linked to raised risk of a mental health problem. This may partly explain why the death rates may be higher in the year after abortion, than the year after having a baby, since depression may lead to suicide.

Red Flag Mental Health Warnings Before Choosing Abortion
Whilst anyone can suffer with their mental health, there are factors that increase the risk of having longer-term emotional problems after an abortion.[7]

Preventing bad mental health resulting from abortion
Previous pregnancy loss is a sensitive issue for many women. If you have had any previous pregnancy loss such as miscarriage, abortion or stillbirth, these are risk factors which may show you need more counselling. Give yourself permission to discuss any sensitive feelings around past loss and discuss any lingering concerns.

Knowing that there is a dose effect – previous losses increase your risk of mental health problems after an abortion – will help you plan.

The following checklist will help you learn whether you are at risk of more severe reactions following abortion.[8]

Checklist of Risk
(adapted from the American Psychological Association, 2008)

If you are considering aborting a pregnancy, be very cautious if any of the following apply:

1. Your pregnancy is wanted or meaningful.

2. You are facing pressure from others to abort.

3. There is opposition to abortion by partners, family or friends.

4. You are unsure and double-minded about the abortion decision.

5. There is lack of social support from others.

6. You have certain personality traits, such as low self-esteem, a pessimistic outlook, feel you have no control over life.

7. You have a history of mental health problems before the pregnancy.

8. You have feelings of shame.

9. You feel the need for secrecy.

10. You are likely to be exposed to anti-abortion pickets or people.

11. You are prone to use of avoidance and denial coping strategies.

12. You have feelings of commitment to the pregnancy.

13. You are not sure that you will have the ability to cope with the abortion.

14. You have had a previous abortion(s).

15. You have had a previous abortion late in pregnancy.

Suicide and Pregnancy Loss

It has been known since the 1990s that unwanted pregnancy itself is a mental health risk. So, will having an abortion lower that risk?

Doctors studied this, and the graphs on the opposite page show their findings.

These bar charts compare suicide attempts before and after abortion with before and after a birth. It shows at a glance what was discovered for every 100,000 women. In order to imagine 100,000 pregnant women, think of a large stadium like Wembley in London full of women. The height of the bars will then give an idea of the numbers of women feeling suicidal or not feeling suicidal in different situations of birth and abortion in that stadium.

These bar charts on suicide attempts are also visible for before and after pregnancy and abortion in Chapter 13 'Teenage Pregnancy and Abortion – Take Special Care'.[10]

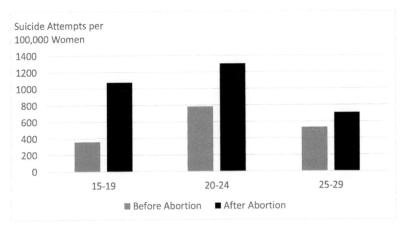

(a) before and after abortion, by age group

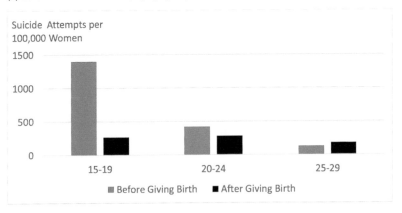

(b) before and after giving birth, by age group

Rate of attempted suicide per 100,000 women (a) before and after abortion or (b) before and after giving birth, for each of the three youngest age groups.
(Source: Suicides after pregnancy. Mental health may deteriorate as a direct effect of induced abortion. Morgan, C L ; Evans, M ; Peters, J R. BMJ (Clinical research ed.), 22 March 1997, Vol.314(7084), pp.902; author reply 902-3.)

Abortion Suicide Attempts
Comparing rate of attempted suicides per 100,000 abortions for before to after the pregnancy ended. These are in three age groups.[9]

While attempted suicide numbers are not the same as completed suicides, the authors of this BMJ study still concluded, 'The increased risk of suicide after an induced abortion may therefore be a consequence of the procedure itself.'

Close Relationship Breakdown After Abortion

While some couples see their abortion was the right thing at the time, there is also evidence that it can affect the relationship badly. The range of potential inter-personal conflicts, reaching to the couple's parents, existing children and subsequent children, is huge. For instance, the woman may have felt she was not given a choice, while on the other hand the man can feel humiliated and bereaved if he did not want to lose his child.

Emotional turmoil in both partners after an abortion can seriously affect close relationships. Although some women and their partners may feel relief and move on, strains between them can develop quickly, or years later. Any breakdown of relationships tends to damage the woman emotionally and financially, just when she is most needing support.

The book *Complications: Abortion's Impact on Women* gives testimonies from women on these issues. For instance, one of 100 conversations collected goes: 'My husband started threatening me with separation if I did not agree to have an abortion . . . He kept yelling at me to sign the papers or abort the baby.' The authors, who include a female surgeon and a female psychologist, conclude: 'Healthcare professionals should be aware of the correlation between abuse and abortion . . . Far from eliminating abuse, obtaining an abortion can actually increase intimate partner violence.'[11]

I have had women in their seventies and eighties come to me and describe the continuing distress they suffer over abortions they had many years ago. Then there was a healthy young man who committed suicide straight after failing to persuade his girlfriend to keep their baby that he had longed for.

Mental and emotional ill health is a risk for any woman and her partner after abortion. It can even strike those who had no doubts at the time of the abortion.

Mortality Concerns After Abortion

Mental health factors, including suicidal feelings after abortion, may partly explain the rise in mortality rates of women in the years following abortion. (See Chapter 17 'Mortality of Women After Birth and Abortion.)

However, help is available. These feelings of anxiety, shame, depression and loss can be helped, and there are a range of support groups, one-to-one counselling and post-abortion programmes around the UK. But this may take time and persistence, and more than one type of professional help. Above all, if you feel you just cannot go on, if you are having suicidal thoughts . . .

RED FLAG

Feeling Suicidal?

If you feel you cannot go on . . . if you have suicidal thoughts

TELL SOMEONE YOU TRUST NOW.

In the UK, dial 111, the NHS doorway to urgent help.

Chapter 20
Infertility After Abortion

This chapter covers:

- What is infertility?

- Risk of infertility after abortion

- Reasons for a woman's future fertility problems after abortion

- What can be done to prevent infertility after abortion?

At the time of an unwanted pregnancy, you may not be concerned with having children at a later stage, yet most people have hopes of a family one day. The health professional's responsibility is to help you weigh up any negative effects the treatment may have on this.

While care for women undergoing abortion has improved, there is evidence that having an abortion may affect future fertility. Most abortions remove a healthy pregnancy; this delays future pregnancy, and with rising age, a delay can reduce the woman's chances of another healthy birth.

So, let's look a bit deeper . . .

What is Infertility?
Infertility is defined by the inability to achieve a pregnancy after 12 months or more regular and unprotected sexual intercourse.[1] Here we include complications linked to abortion which can lead to being unable to deliver a healthy baby. This includes early miscarriage linked to the previous abortion. Overall, infertility affects about 1 in 7 couples[2] (3.5 million British people) and in a third of instances the problem is related to the woman.

Risk of Infertility After Abortion

There are various reasons why a previous abortion could give a woman problems conceiving and delivering safely at term. But what does research say about the overall risk when all these factors are brought together?

According to a British study in 2005, women who have had an abortion are *7 times* more likely to have trouble conceiving than those who haven't.[3] A study from Shanghai in the *Journal of Obstetrics and Gynaecology 2001* noted a significant association between fertility and previous abortion.[4] A Greek study showed abortion as an independent and significant risk to future fertility, with the risk increasing after a second abortion.[5]

Reasons for a Woman's Future Fertility Problems After Abortion

1. **She cannot conceive again** (known as subfecundity). After an abortion, women are 7 times more likely to be unable to conceive again.[6]

2. **She suffers surgical damage to the cervix** (neck of the womb), as the cervical channel is widened. This can weaken the ability of the cervix to hold the fetus in the womb. The Royal College of Obstetricians and Gynaecologists puts the risk of damage at up to 1 in 100 surgical abortions,[7] but it may be a large underestimate.

3. **Early miscarriage.** Cervical damage and retained products of conception may be part of the reason for early miscarriages linked to abortion. The incidence of miscarriage increases if a woman conceives again within three months of the abortion.[8] This would suggest it is better to delay conception longer than longer months after an abortion.

4. **Infection of the womb and fallopian tubes.**[9] Following an abortion, there is a greater risk of infection of the womb and fallopian tubes. Infection can block the tubes, which reduces the chances of conceiving another child.

FALLOPIAN TUBE OBSTRUCTION

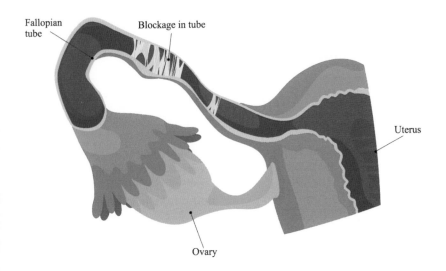

Fallopian tube

Blockage in tube

Uterus

Ovary

5. **Ectopic pregnancy.** Ectopic pregnancy, where the fertilised egg implants itself outside of the womb, has been linked to previous abortion. Sadly, ectopic pregnancies cannot survive and must be removed to protect the woman. An Australian study in 2006 found that a woman's risk of ectopic pregnancy rises 7– 10 times after female infection and Pelvic Inflammatory Disease (PID)[10] – and an Indian study put it at 6 times higher.[11] The sequence can be that abortion leads to the pelvic infection which then goes on to become PID, leading to an ectopic pregnancy. One in 10 women who have PID will have an ectopic pregnancy, according to a study in 2006.[12]

6. **Stillbirth.** Unfortunately, when an abortion leads to infection, the risk of stillbirth in a follow-on pregnancy (when the baby dies before or during birth) is nearly 5 times higher, according to a Scandinavian study in 2003.[13] How could this happen? It seems that low-grade infection may be introduced by surgery at the time of the abortion, where it lies quietly undetected. Then at the next pregnancy, the germs multiply fast and are transmitted to the baby as a fatal infection.[14]

NORMAL PREGNANCY   ECTOPIC PREGNANCY

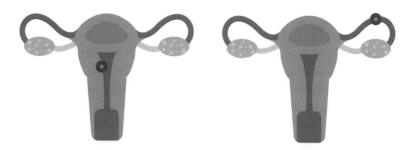

7. **The risk of placenta praevia** rises after one or more induced abortions. This is when the placenta is lying too low in the womb and can bleed through the cervix into the vagina. That bleeding means the baby must be delivered early to save the mother, so the baby may be very premature, with all the problems that brings.[15] (More on this in Chapter 21 'Premature Birth After Abortion'.)

Of 101 women who told their abortion story, some reported infertility due to a damaged cervix (neck of the womb) or badly scarred uterus (womb). Of the 40 who answered the question on infertility, 23% reported that despite their best efforts they were unable to have children.[16]

What Can be Done to Prevent Infertility After Abortion?
Abortions done with the greatest care cannot eliminate all chance of these complications. If you are going ahead, then before and after abortion inform your doctor of any unpleasant-smelling discharge from the vagina or heavy bleeding.

Afterwards, seek treatment promptly for any signs of infection such as fever, sweats, fainting and nausea, as they could be life-threatening sepsis, as well as seriously affecting your fertility. 'Antibiotics are commonly given to women before induced abortion, but they are not always effective.'[17]

Other evidence
In 2013, a large team of researchers in North America, after 10 years' work, concluded that 'Evidence linking infertility to previous induced abortion is overwhelming.'[18]

You may feel confused by the conflicting views on infertility but ultimately it is *your* health and *your* choice.

Chapter 21
Premature Birth After Abortion
by Professor J. Wyatt

This chapter covers:

- What is a premature birth?

- Why is preterm birth dangerous?

- What factors increase the risk of preterm delivery?

- Very preterm birth – extra dangers

- Why should abortion raise the risk of later preterm delivery?

- The main message

What is a Premature Birth?
A normal pregnancy lasts about 9 months or 40 weeks. When birth occurs before 37 weeks, it is defined technically as 'preterm' or in popular speech 'premature' or 'prem' for short. In the UK, about 7% of all births occur before 37 weeks. Previous abortion has a strong statistical link with preterm birth in subsequent pregnancies.

Why is Preterm Birth Dangerous?
The more preterm a baby is at the time of birth, the more likely they are to have problems in the first days and weeks of life, because of immaturity of the organs. Babies born before 32 weeks account for about 1% of all births in the UK. These are known as 'very preterm'. These babies are likely to require treatment in hospital for weeks and, sadly, they have an increased

risk of complications, particularly immature lungs and brain. Brain injury is a major concern because it may have long-term effects which can include cerebral palsy, learning and educational difficulties, and behavioural problems, including autistic spectrum disorder.

The greatest risk is with babies born at the limits of continuing life – that is, born at around 23–25 weeks. The numbers are relatively small (about 2 per 1,000 births in the UK) but unfortunately, these babies have a high risk of death in the period immediately after birth. Between 20% and 50% of babies born alive will die before discharge from hospital, and those who survive have a high risk (up to 50%) of some form of permanent brain injury.[1],[2]

Does previous abortion have a strong statistical link with preterm birth in the next pregnancies?

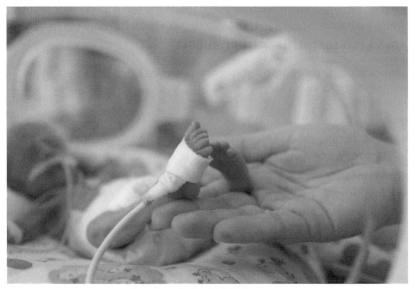

Premature baby in intensive care

What Factors Increase the Risk of Preterm Delivery?
Many studies have been carried out to find what increases the risk that a mother will have a preterm delivery, and several factors have been identified. These include medical issues such as various forms of infection, abnormalities of the womb and cervix, and high maternal blood pressure; and social factors such as social deprivation and domestic abuse.

A strong and consistent link has been found between a previous induced abortion and an increased risk of preterm delivery in a subsequent pregnancy. There is a 30%–60% increased risk of preterm delivery following a previous induced abortion.

There are statistical methods for adjusting the figures to take into account known risk factors for prematurity. Considering the other conditions like those listed above, a study combining 37 other studies found that one previous induced abortion made a preterm birth 27% more likely. Two or more previous abortions made preterm birth 62% more likely.[3] Another study of studies published in 2016 found a greater increased risk after two or more abortions using the surgical method.[4]

It's important to understand what these studies are showing – that the more abortions a woman has, the more likely it is that she will have a premature baby from a later pregnancy. Harvard University researchers found that Black American women with more than one prior induced abortion double their future premature delivery risk compared to Black American women without prior abortions.[5]

So, it is fair to say that there is a strong scientific link, backed up by statistics, between abortion and preterm delivery of a baby later in life.

Very Preterm Birth – Extra Dangers

Studies have also shown that the risk of 'very preterm' delivery (below 32 weeks) is significantly increased when there has been a previous induced abortion. A study of 12 different studies in 2009 found that women who'd had one or more previous induced abortions had on average a *64% higher risk* of a very preterm delivery compared to women with no previous abortions.[6] As we have seen, it is the most premature babies who are sadly at the most risk of dying or of long-term and permanent after-effects.[7]

The scientific evidence of a causal link between previous induced abortion and increased risk of preterm delivery appears to be very robust and consistent. The effect is consistent across studies published over a 50-year period from the 1960s to the present. It is consistent in studies involving many different countries with widely differing socioeconomic backgrounds and widely differing attitudes towards induced abortion.

Why Should Abortion Raise the Risk of Later Preterm Delivery?

Several known biological factors can explain the link between abortion and subsequent preterm delivery. For instance, there is strong evidence that induced abortion increases the risk of complications from infection in a later pregnancy, and it is well known that pelvic infection and chronic pelvic inflammatory disease (PID) increase the risk of subsequent preterm delivery.[8] This may be the result of hidden infection caused by surgery at the time of the abortion. Surgical abortion may injure the cervix making it vulnerable to infection. This sort of damage to the cervix (leading to the condition known as 'cervical incompetence') is a well-known cause of subsequent preterm delivery.

It is possible that surgical instruments inserted through the cervix at abortion may increase the risk of damage to the endometrium (the lining of the womb), which may interfere with normal positioning of the placenta in a later pregnancy. This would increase the risk of a condition called *placenta praevia*, in which the placenta is abnormally placed leading to an increased risk of serious bleeding during the pregnancy. This is well known as a risk factor for preterm delivery.

Studies have shown a consistent statistical relationship between induced abortion and subsequent preterm delivery due to infection or cervical problems, but not between abortion and preterm delivery resulting from other factors like high blood pressure in the mother. This provides further support for what we suspect – that it is the abortion itself which is adding to the increased risk of having a preterm baby in a later pregnancy.[9]

The Main Message

Most people are unaware of this clear connection between induced abortion and an increased risk of preterm delivery in follow-on pregnancies. Based on published data, approximately 14% of all women in UK who deliver have already had an abortion.[10] So using this figure and an increased risk of 30% of very preterm birth, it can be calculated that previous abortion is leading to *several hundred extra* very preterm infants being born at less than 32 weeks every year, and more than 100 extra very preterm infants born below 28 weeks.

Approximately half of all abortions in England and Wales are undertaken in women under the age of 25 years, whereas 75% of all live births occur in mothers over the age of 25. Most of the women who are considering abortion will later deliver one or more children. It is *essential* that women and their partners are adequately informed about the possible effects of abortion on them and follow-on pregnancies.

In 2007, a group of researchers estimated that in the United States in one year alone, prior induced abortions led to more than 1,000 cases of cerebral palsy because of babies being born prematurely.[11]

Conclusions
One abortion significantly raises the woman's risk of premature birth in the next or later pregnancies. Repeat abortions means a higher risk for her and her family of this serious complication. It is this group of infants that are sadly most likely to die in the first days and weeks after birth. And in those who survive, there is a significant risk of brain damage leading to cerebral palsy and behavioural problems.

Appendix 1
ABC of Spiritual Beliefs on Pregnancy & Abortion

This appendix covers:

- Your worldview

- An A B C of worldviews for pregnancy and abortion: Atheism, Buddhism, Christianity, Hindu, Islam, Judaism and Sikhism

- To be human is to make mistakes

Pregnancy and abortion raise spiritual questions such as, when does life begin . . . and end? Why do some people afterwards feel regret or that they made a mistake? Why do some feel shame or fear? Some people go through pregnancy and abortion and feel fine. But stories from pastors, doctors and counsellors show that some feel very differently and have deep questions.

This appendix will help you reflect on these questions by explaining the position of major faiths (including atheism as a 'belief') and what help they offer.

Health professionals know that spirituality can benefit health and decisions. The General Medical Council affirms the importance of the medical professional understanding the individual's worldview.

Medical professor Richard Vincent (previously Dean of Brighton Medical School) reminds people that, out of 1,200 scientific studies of individuals, 81% show benefit from faith in healthcare and just 4% harm.[1]

Your Worldview

When you read the Making Choices chapters you thought about your heart beliefs. While science brings benefits in the physical world, it is not equipped for questions of the heart. These deep beliefs make up our 'worldview' and steer many of our choices in life.

What's your Worldview?

Your worldview is your basic belief about where you came from, why you are here and what happens to you when you die. It is your view of the world, morality and the universe.

Life and its choices are easier when spiritual beliefs agree with instinctive human values which some people call our 'conscience'. Philosopher Jonathan Haidt has studied the values found in all cultures and discovered that care for others, freedom and justice (fairness) are some of the strongest.[2]

An A B C of Worldviews on Pregnancy and Abortion

Here in brief is how the common belief systems handle such issues.

ATHEISM

Atheists believe there is no creator God, lesser gods or any spiritual dimension. Some believe in the basic goodness of humanity.

The 2011 British census found 29,267 people declared themselves atheists out of 57 million people in the UK.

Some atheists are strongly against abortion, such as pro-life humanists,[3] while for others free abortion has been promoted widely and intensively.

On the question 'When does life begin?' atheist views vary widely. The following got high votes online:

> 'Life is an unbroken strand from parent to offspring. Sure, a microscopic blastocyst [human embryo] is alive, but so were the sperm and egg that it came from. There's no point at which life "began".'[4]

Some humanists use this argument to oppose abortion. They say:

> 'Humanists have a long history of being a secular voice of social justice and we affirm the Universal Declaration of Human Rights as granted in Article 3 should apply to even the youngest and least developed members of our species ... And we refuse to discriminate against those conceived through the violence of rape.'[5]

Utilitarianism, a form of atheism is 'An ethical philosophy in which the happiness of the greatest number of people in the society is considered the greatest good. According to this philosophy, an action is morally right if its consequences lead to happiness (absence of pain), and wrong if it ends in unhappiness (pain).'[6]

It seems most NHS and private abortion clinics are 'utilitarian' in practice. It's as if they are saying, 'You can do what you like with your pregnancy as long as it will make you happy.' There seems scant awareness that happiness and feeling 'right' may not be the result. At times, it's a sort of practical atheism. In general, health staff involved in abortion seem to hold the view, 'If you want an abortion, we will do one.'

Expected result versus the reality. This utilitarian approach can throw up conflicts when the reality after making a choice of action is different from expected: for instance if you expected to feel happier but end up less happy. Or you expected a short, simple solution but in real life, the result is anything but simple and sorted. Or you expected to be out of pain and shame, but the result is distress, guilt and regret. Or you expected most close relationships to be fine now, so why are they falling apart?

BUDDHISM

The legend of the Buddha born around 586 BCE is the core of the religion. Buddhist sources are the sacred texts and the way to enlightenment by following the Noble Eightfold Path. A central conviction is that one should cause no harm to others. Salvation is by outward practices and special medication. Ethical conduct includes: 1. Take no life. 2. Abstain from sexual misconduct.[7]

Buddhists regard human life as beginning at conception. For this reason, many are opposed to abortion and the morning-after pill. In everyday practice, Buddhists, like those of other faiths, show wide variation in where they draw the line on unwanted pregnancy.

'Japanese Buddhist tradition includes the mizuko kuyo ritual for post pregnancy loss, which requires a full apology from the parents to make amends to an aborted child.'[8]

'Of course, abortion, from a Buddhist viewpoint, is an act of killing and is negative, generally speaking. But it depends on the circumstances. If the unborn child will be retarded or if the birth will create serious problems for the parent, these are cases where there can be an exception. I think abortion should be approved or disapproved according to each circumstance.'

Dalai Lama, *New York Times*, 28/11/1993[9]

'Buddhists face a difficulty where an abortion is medically necessary to save the life of the mother and so a life will be lost whether there is or isn't an abortion. In such cases the moral status of an abortion will depend on the intentions of those carrying it out.'[10]

We were not able to find offers of face-to-face pregnancy counselling by Buddhists, but more general counselling can be found online.

CHRISTIANITY

Christians believe in one Creator God. Their main authorities are the Holy Bible and the life and teaching of Jesus Christ. Most Christians say the Bible teaches that human life begins at conception, quoting passages like 'you knit me together in my mother's womb' (Psalm 139, verse 13) and 'from the time my mother conceived me' (Psalm 51, verse 5).[11]

So human life is beyond value, before and after birth because humans, both female and male, are made in the image of God – an imperfect but priceless reflection of God himself (Genesis chapter 1, verses 26–27). Human values like truth and love, justice and care, are showing the mother and father heart of the God who Jesus Christ called 'Father'. So abortion is viewed by most Bible teachers as taking human life and that the consequences include separation from God now and in the next life . . . unless the offer of the way back to God is taken up.

There *is* a way back. To show this, Christians may point to the famous story told by Jesus Christ about a father who welcomes back his shame-faced child with open arms (known as the 'Prodigal Son' in Luke's gospel chapter 11, verses 11–32).

Christian leaders usually support abortion if the mother's life is in danger. The thinking is that if nothing is done, then two lives will be lost. A common example of this is an ectopic pregnancy, where the fetus must be removed to save the mother's life.

Historically, Christians transformed Roman society by caring for unwanted girls and weak babies instead of leaving them exposed outside to die.[12] They opposed abortion, as did pagan doctors like Hippocrates in 400 BC. Many churches, following the way of Jesus, welcome and support single mothers and unmarried couples with pregnancies and children.

Abortion remains largely unspoken about in churches, but some are recognising this and striving to be humble, non-judgemental and welcoming. They may point to Christ's dramatic intervention to help the shame and danger of a woman caught in bed with a man not her husband; he saved her from being stoned (John's gospel chapter 8, verses 1– 11).

For more help, see 'Appendix 2: Finding Help'.

HINDUISM
The guiding books for Hinduism are called the Vedas. For many Hindus, religion is more about what you do and what you believe. Hindus believe in a universal soul or God called Brahman. This God can take on many forms as gods or goddesses. Hindus believe in reincarnation – belief that the soul is eternal and lives many lifetimes, sometimes in a human body, sometimes in an animal body.

Hinduism is generally opposed to abortion, except where it is necessary to save the mother's life. Hindus believe in the principle of 'ahimsa' (non-violence), choosing the action that will do least harm to all involved.[13]

Hindu pregnancy and abortion counselling seems hard to find in the UK, from our own research.

ISLAM
In Islam, The Holy Qur'an and the teaching of the Prophet Mohammed are the main source of authority for worship and living. 'Whoever saves a life,

it is as though he had saved the life of all mankind . . .' (Qur'an chapter 5, verse 32). Muslims believe in one God called Allah. His commands are to be obeyed in all matters of life. The final future of the human is weighed at the Judgement on a balance of right and wrong acts performed in their earthly life.

'All schools of Muslim law accept that abortion is permitted if continuing the pregnancy would put the mother's life in real danger. This is the only reason accepted for abortion after 120 days of the pregnancy.'[14]

Talking to Muslim doctors throughout my 40-year career, all without exception have taken conception as the beginning of the individual human. Marriage and family are considered to be the basic social unit of Islamic society.[15] Secrecy and fear of family backlash may put a pregnant Muslim woman or teenager in a difficult, even a dangerous place, especially if a baby has been conceived outside marriage. Strong codes of professional confidentiality should ensure the safety of those who seek pregnancy advice.

Shaleena says . . .

'Religiously I am a Muslim. For us abortion is an unforgivable sin. Now I am excluded from salvation.'[16]

Specifically Muslim crisis pregnancy and post-abortion counselling is not easily found in the UK, although thousands of Muslims work as NHS professionals in the UK and will understand the Muslim worldview.

JUDAISM

The Jews have a saying, 'The one who saves a life saved the whole world.' The Jewish holy book is the Tanakh, basically the same as the Old Testament in the Christian Bible. They believe there is one God. The final eternal future of each human is weighed at the Judgement on the balance of right and wrong actions in the earthly life, in obedience to the laws of the Tanakh. Jews have often defended the unborn since ancient times, while giving priority to preserving the life of the mother over the child.

In 2015, the *Jewish Journal* reported that roughly half of modern American

Jews, whether Liberal or Orthodox, say abortion should be permissible in all cases. However, this cannot be supported by the Tanakh, nor the traditions and values of Judaism.

SIKHISM

If you treat everyone with utmost respect, perhaps you will be led to God during your human incarnation. Sikhs believe in one God and that death leads to reincarnation as a human or an animal. The Sikh sacred text, the Guru Granth Sahib, says that the body is just clothing for the soul and is discarded at death.[17] Ethics: Tobacco, stealing and adultery are forbidden.

Sikhs believe there is one God who is both present in all things and everyone; they support the equality of all men and women.[18] Sikhs regard life as starting at conception and many do not believe that lifestyle abortions are justified.

To be Human is to Make Mistakes

So, it appears that most of the world's faiths, including some atheists, value unborn human life highly. What do they offer people feeling regret and sensing they have made mistakes?

It seems religions vary widely over what happens to those who have regrets. Can guilt be removed? Can mental peace return?

In my experience, and that of the counsellor who helped write this book, yes, there is a way forward – there is hope. Like for that old lady who visibly relaxed, smiled and sighed with relief when she heard 'Yes,' in answer to her question, 'Can God ever forgive me for the abortion?'

You can research many faiths. I found Jesus Christ offers a solid promise: God accepts those who come to him with genuine regrets; in fact, God as 'Father' longs to welcome anyone who turns to Jesus Christ (see John's gospel chapter 3, verse 16).

Christians point out how Jesus promised a criminal who asked for help during his execution, 'today you will be with me in paradise' (see Luke's gospel chapter 23, verse 43).[19]

Jesus also said, 'whoever comes to me I will never drive away' (see John's gospel chapter 6, verse 37). Countless people record that their regrets, shame and anxiety were swept clean by Christ who gave them a fresh start.[20]

Appendix 2
Finding Help
For Pregnancy, For Pregnant Teenagers, For Parenting, For Adoption, Post Abortion and For Pregnancy Screening and Fetus Disability

Online counselling is popular now because it's more private. Many of the following sites offer this.

TEENAGE PREGNANCY HELP

- **Pregnancy Choices Directory** at http://www.pregnancychoicesdirectory. com/ will point you to an advice centre near you. Free pregnancy testing is offered from this site. Advice centres are all over the UK.

- **The GP, family planning clinic and school nurse** are there for you, but beware they may hurry you down the abortion route whether you have thought it over or not. (See Chapter 13 'Teenage Pregnancy'.)

- **The Mix** http://www.themix.org.uk/get-support/speak-to-our-team? The Mix is a UK-based charity that provides free, confidential support for young people under 25 via online, social media and mobile.

- **Relate for children and young people** https://www.relate.org.uk/ relationship-help/help-children-and-young-people

- **NHS choices** http://www.nhs.uk/conditions/pregnancy-and-baby/ pages/teenager-pregnant.aspx#

- In Northern Ireland **Love for Life** helps young people value themselves, relationships and sex. Teens can text questions to a team of doctors about any aspect of sexual health or relationships at http://www. oscarandmartha.com. Telephone 02838 820555.

HELP FOR TEENAGE PARENTS

- **Gingerbread** https://gingerbread.org.uk/content/681/Teenage-parents-benefits-finder#

PARENTING HELP IN THE UK

- **Love for Life** offers parents practical tips and support http://www.loveforlife.org.uk/sectors/parents/

- **Finances, housing, benefits** and so on look at end of Chapter 8, 'Parenting Explored'.

- **Single parenting** look at end of Chapter 8, 'Parenting Explored'.

HELP FOR PARENTS OF PREGNANT TEENAGERS

- J. Jeffes, *Unplanned Pregnancy: Talking with Teenagers* (Hove: Lean Press, 2013). This short booklet is full of practical advice for parents of teenagers and worth reading before a problem pregnancy enters the family.

ADOPTION HELP IN THE UK

- **Coram**, the UK children's charity, has over 40 years' experience in finding children families to take them for life. It is one of the largest agencies in the UK. http://www.coramadoption.org.uk/about-adoption. Phone 020 7421 2600.

- **Adoption Matters** have been helping children find their future for 70 years.

- **ASIST** (Adoption Support in Society Today) started in Somerset in 1993 as a support group for families who had adopted children. ASIST works to support children, birth parents and adoptive parents. ASIST runs a national helpline and receives adoption enquiries from across the country. It is not involved in the actual adoption process but they will discuss the subject in confidence with anyone who wants to know more. The charity will also act as a 'signpost', referring callers to appropriate voluntary or professional organisations in their area where they can get practical help. You may wish to contact them before contacting social services which vary across the country. http://www.babyadoptionasist.co.uk. Helpline: 01823 282351.

- **Social Services.** You can contact any local Social Services department within your Local Authority.

- **Adoption UK** Is a useful government site outlining the adoption or fostering process, birth parents' rights, fathers' rights and links to other useful sites. https://www.adoptionuk.org

- **Government website** https://www.gov.uk/child-adoption/birth-parents-your-rights is a useful section for birth parents from the help site above.

- **Family Lives**, formerly Parentline, is for stepparents and other parents and has been around since 1999. They have a large staff working for separated families, stepparents and parents in prison. http://www.familylives.org.uk.

HELP WITH DEBT
- Debt IVA for debts over £5,000 http://www.debtiva.co.uk

- National Debt Help http://www.national-debt-help.com

MENTAL HEALTH SUPPORT AFTER PREGNANCY LOSS FROM ABORTION OR MISCARRIAGE

> If you feel you cannot go on . . . if you have suicidal ideas . . .
>
> **TELL SOMEONE YOU TRUST NOW.**
>
> Dial 111, the NHS doorway to urgent psychiatric help.

When you suffer the loss of something close to you the shock and grief can feel overwhelming. With emotional issues after abortion, it's better to share your feelings with someone you can trust, such as your local family doctor or a local pastor. Talk it over with other women who have been through loss, and your partner if possible.

POST-ABORTION COUNSELLING
Post-abortion counselling is available near most UK cities. Search online for one of the many post-abortion counselling services across the UK. Many will charge nothing.

- **Rachel's Vineyard** has centres in European countries, UK and USA. http://www.rachelsvineyard.org.uk/contact-us.

- **We Are Open** is an abortion recovery course which is run by experienced Christian professionals. We Are Open runs healing weekends and other resources for individuals and gives guidance to churches in the UK wanting to get into post-abortion care. http://www.weareopen.org.uk.

- **Image** in Manchester offers a pregnancy helpline for support before and after abortion to people of all faiths or none and for those in prison. http://pregnancyhelpline.co.uk. Phone 0333 772 0237. Text 07797 803 693. Image runs an acclaimed training course for counsellors.

COPING WITH BEREAVEMENT AFTER PREGNANCY LOSS

If you feel anxious and depressed after stillbirth, pregnancy loss or abortion loss the following can also help:

- **Cruse Bereavement Care** http://www.crusebereavementcare.org.uk/useful-links.

- **Mind** https://www.mind.org.uk.

- **Depression Alliance** merged with mind in 2016 https://www.mind.org.uk/about-us/what-we-do/depression-alliance.

- **Mental Health Foundation** has its own list of help sites https://www.mentalhealth.org.uk/your-mental-health/getting-help.

Stories of people's experiences

Finding how other people felt and coped can be a real step to freeing you from isolation and low feelings. Perhaps sharing your own story can bring your feelings out as a step on the journey of healing. http://www.pregnancychoicesdirectory.com/peoplesstories/abortion/ 2932/keep-the-baby-or-have-a-termination.

HELPS FOR FETUS DISABILITY AND PREGNANCY SCREENING ISSUES

- **NHS Choices** antenatal screening tests in pregnancy http://www.nhs.uk/Conditions/Pages/hub.aspx.

- **ARC** (Antenatal Results and Choices) offers emotional support and non-directive counselling for people facing pain after hard pregnancy choices and provides a range of literature and information http://www.arc-uk.org/.

- **A Heartbreaking Choice** is 'lovingly dedicated to all who have made a heartbreaking choice'. It covers major and minor fetus problems. There are sections for spirituality and religious leaders, with stories of people coping with disability http://www.aheartbreakingchoice.com.

- Your Personal physician, GP and medical services.

FAITH-BASED SOURCES OF HELP

Pregnancy counselling services, for both before, during and after abortion, are available all over the UK. Some have no faith basis and others are run by Christians but are open to people of any faith or none. The same applies in North America, Israel and Australasia. This list points to the largest only:

- **Rachel's Vineyard – UK and Ireland** is a safe place to renew and rebuild your life after abortion. The healing weekends offer you a supportive, confidential and non-judgemental environment where women and men can deal with painful post-abortion emotions.

National calls UK 07505 904 656 (Marene)

Midlands: 07734 059 080 (Rachel)

South East: 07851 331 816 (Pam)

South West: 07900 734 207 (Sona)

Scotland: 07816 942 824 (Andrea)

http://www.rachelsvineyard.org.uk/contact-us

Ireland: 087 859 2877

http://www.facebook.com/RVIreland/

http://www.rachelsvineyard.ie/

- **Pregnancy Choices Directory** covers the UK. It points to help centres for those facing unplanned pregnancy or after abortion http://www.pregnancychoicesdirectory.com/.

- **Image Pregnancy Helpline** covers the Greater Manchester Area offering support before and after abortion to people of all faiths or none http://www.pregnancyhelpline.co.uk/. Phone 0333 772 0237. Text 07797 803 693.

- **Jewish pregnancy and post-abortion counselling services** are not common but can be accessed through http://www.Jewishtherapists.co.uk.

- **Jewish counselling services: Raphael, the Jewish Counselling Service** http://www.jvn.org.uk/raphael-the-jewish-counselling-service-134.php.

- **Jewish Bereavement Counselling Service** https://childbereavementuk.org/database/7369/jewish-bereavement-counselling-service/

- **Pregnancy Matters at Life** is a UK charity offering pregnancy counselling and practical help with housing and baby clothes. They can be contacted by text, message or national helpline 0808 802 5433 https://lifecharity.org.uk/.

- **Call the local church minister, Iman or other spiritual helper** or helpline by searching under local churches, mosques and places of worship.

- **UCB prayer line** offers a trained and confidential talk with prayer from a Christian with people of any faith or none. Ring 0845 456 7729 in the UK or 1890 940 300 in the Republic of Ireland http://www.ucb.co.uk/prayerline.

- **Sikh pregnancy and post-abortion counselling** is not easily found in the UK. Sikhs like their stillborn babies to be given respect in burial by cremation.

HELP IF YOU HAVE REGRETS AFTER ABORTION

- **Freedom in Christ**. If you still feel imprisoned by regrets, think of joining a small group on the award-winning Freedom in Christ course http://www.ficm.org.uk/.

- **The Post-Abortion Healing Course** (written for Christians) is held at Holy Trinity Brompton, London and other churches in the UK. For details of the next course go to https://www.htb.org/whats-on/courses/post-abortion-healingAu17 or contact courses@htb.org.uk or call 020 7052 0323 for further information.

- **The Step by Step Support Programme** is a course for recovery from any form of child loss. Run by Image in Manchester (charity number 1141832) it has been developed as a resource for Christian pregnancy centres in the UK, and mainly facilitates post-abortion support. However, many centres also support clients after miscarriage, stillbirth, child loss and those in prison separated from their children. For details of pregnancy and post-abortion counselling go to http://www.image. org.uk or http://www.pregnancyhelpline.co.uk/ or contact office@ imagenet.org.uk or call 0161 273 8090.

- **Other faith-based counselling services** are available in many major towns in the UK. Many GP surgeries have Christians or those of other faiths on the staff. Churches have ministers, hospitals and prisons have chaplains, mosques, synagogues and other places of worship will often supply advice and counsel that can be found by phone call or by searching the web.

- **Counselling Directory** is a comprehensive database of UK counsellors and psychotherapists, with information on their training, experience and fees http://www.counselling-directory.org.uk/.

OVERSEAS
In Israel/Palestine

Pregnancy counselling and practical help for mums and babies can be found at http://www.beadchaim.com.

In the USA, Canada, Spain, Holland, Italy and France

- **Rachel's Vineyard:** call our toll-free national hotlines: 877 HOPE 4 ME (877 467 3463). National Hotline for Abortion Recovery: 866 482 LIFE (866-482-5433).

- **After Abortion** offers telephone and email advice both before and after abortion. Toll-free helpline: 1 866 482 5433. http://www.afterabortion. org/help-healing.

Appendix 3
Glossary

Abortion: the intentional ending of a pregnancy with the death of the unborn so that the baby is not born alive.

Anaesthetic: medicines or injections to make you numb or sleepy so that painful procedures or surgery can be done.

Antenatal care: care of you and your fetus up to and after birth.

Anxiety: an unpleasant sense of fear that something is threatening you. It is often linked with depression and low mood.

Bereavement, grieving: feeling sorrowful and mourning the death and loss of a loved one.

Cervix: a tightly closed muscle around a small hole at the top of the vagina. It is the gateway to the womb for the man's sperm to reach the egg. It's the outlet for the baby to be born through, or for the aborted foetus to be taken out through.

Cervical incompetence: when the cervix is weakened for some reason, so that it cannot keep the fetus securely in the womb. One human cause of this can be previous stretching through surgical abortion.

Conscience: a person's inner sense of right and wrong which can guide choices and actions.

Conscientious objection: the right of an individual to do or not to do something because of their inner convictions about what is right or wrong, good or harmful. This can apply to them or their action for someone else.

The British abortion law upholds the rights of healthcare staff to have conscientious objection against taking part in abortion.

Consent: when a patient gives permission to someone else to interfere with their body by a medical procedure.

Contraception: attempts to prevent pregnancy by natural or artificial means like the pill, coil, and barriers such as condoms; it may include methods that destroy young embryos in early pregnancy.

Contractions: the periodic tightening and relaxing of the womb which can feel like cramping around the back or abdomen.

Counsellor: a professional who sees a person privately to help them explore what is best for them according to their circumstances, feelings and conscience.

Depression: a feeling and illness like heaviness, darkness and loss of hope which affects your ability to live properly and often comes with anxiety as well. In severe depression, you may feel like ending your life.

Disenfranchised grief: the grief of bereavement which cannot be shown easily to friends, family or in public because of the feeling that one is not meant to be grieving. Abortion can provoke disenfranchised grief; that's because abortion is usually done in the belief it should solve a problem not create a new problem of major loss.

Ectopic pregnancy: when a young human embryo is not growing in the right place, in the womb, but somewhere else. This brings the risk of bursting and bleeding internally.

Embryo: a young human from conception (fertilization) up to 8 weeks of pregnancy, at which point he/she is known as a fetus or baby till birth.

Ethical: something that is morally right. Unethical means it is morally wrong.

Fetal abnormality and disability: when there is a physical or genetic disease in the fetus.

Fetus: the medical name for the unborn baby in the womb from the 8th week of pregnancy until birth.

General anaesthetic: the procedure to put you into a deep sleep using powerful medicines so that painful procedures can be done.

Gestation: the age of the pregnancy or fetus in weeks since the last menstrual period.

Haemorrhage: severe bleeding that can threaten life and may need blood transfusion. Possible causes for the purposes of this book include all types of abortion, infection after abortion and childbirth.

Heart area: anything that reflects someone's deeply held values.

Infertility: when a couple or a woman cannot conceive a baby or bring a pregnancy to a successful live birth.

Labour: the woman's process of delivering her fetus at a birth (or it can be at an abortion).

Local anaesthetic: a medicine usually given by injection to numb part of the body to pain.

Mammogram: a special x-ray of the breast which can detect early breast cancer.

Medical abortion: abortion induced by hormones and chemicals given by mouth, in the vagina or through a vein. Also called 'Pill Abortion'.

Menstrual cycle: the woman's natural process of monthly bleeding when not pregnant. It is preparing your body for pregnancy each month.

Midwife: a specialist to help women through pregnancy, birth and recovery from birth. Most midwives have resisted involvement in abortion.

Miscarriage: the spontaneous loss of a fetus which is too young to survive outside the womb.

Moral: behaviour and choices which are ethically correct according to one's inner convictions or the teaching of great religious leaders.

NHS: The National Health Service of Great Britain.

Oestrogen (Estrogen): a female hormone released in large amounts throughout pregnancy. In a first pregnancy, it changes breast tissue from a cancer safer state before conception to a cancer risky state in early pregnancy. This change is permanent unless the pregnancy continues to 32 weeks – at this point on the breasts become more cancer resistant for life.

PID (Pelvic Inflammatory Disease): a persisting and painful illness of the pelvis following infection, commonly due to chlamydia nowadays.

Prem: short for premature birth.

Premature birth: giving birth before 37 weeks' gestation.

Preterm: means the same as premature.

Preterm labour: is when the woman's uterus contracts and causes the baby to be born prematurely at an age younger than 37 weeks' gestation.

RCOG: is the Royal College of Obstetricians and Gynaecologists.

Screening: testing people to see if there is a disease present. This includes breast cancer screening for older women and screening tests in pregnancy on the mother and fetus.

Sepsis: overwhelming infection which threatens life.

STI: this is short for Sexually Transmitted Infection such as chlamydia.

Suicide: the intentional taking of your own life.

Surgical abortion: ending the pregnancy by sucking out the womb, scraping out the womb or surgical destruction and removal of the fetus from the womb.

Ultrasound scan: a painless and harmless way of looking at the fetus from very early pregnancy until birth.

Uterus: womb.

Womb: the organ in the woman's pelvis, the shape and size of a pear in the non-pregnant woman. It is where healthy fetuses grow until birth.

My Notes

Here you can jot down thoughts, feelings and questions you may have.

It will help to take these along to an appointment with a health professional or clinic.

My past medical history:
- My personal doctor

- My past medical history – illnesses, operations, treatments, drugs and food allergies, medication, STI's, contraception, steroids, prescription medicines, supplements not prescribed by a doctor.

My Questions to ask at the clinic:

1.

2.

3.

My Notes

My Notes

Endnotes

PART 1: THE JOURNEY TO A DECISION
Chapter 1: Am I Pregnant?
1. See more in NHS Choices at http://www.nhs.uk/chq/pages/948.aspx?Category-ID=54&SubCategoryID=127 (accessed 07-08-17).
2. See more in NHS Choices at http://www.nhs.uk/chq/pages/948.aspx?Category-ID=54&SubCategoryID=127 (accessed 07-08-17).
3. http://www.babymed.com/positive-pregnancy-test-how-early-after-implantation (accessed 23/2/17).

PART 2: EXPLORING YOUR OPTIONS
Chapter 7: Pregnancy Development Week by Week
1. Female reproductive system, Shutterstock 370633820.
2. I based this on the biological arguments in the article J.K. Findlay et al, 'Human embryo: a biological definition', *Human Reproduction* 22 (Apr 2007): pp. 905–11 found at: https://academic.oup.com/humrep/article-abstract/22/4/905/695880/Human-embryo-a-biological-definition (accessed 26/9/17).
3. http://www.babymed.com/positive-pregnancy-test-how-early-after-implantation (accessed 23/2/17.
4. *The Telegraph,* 27 April 2016. http://www.telegraph.co.uk/content/dam/science/2016/04/26/egg4-large_trans_NvBQzQNjv4Bq5dd29MwfFMR1mtn-yLmH6GudXaa_GsEOdIoFCLIfBGyE.PNG. Also http://www.telegraph.co.uk/science/2016/04/26/bright-flash-of-light-marks-incredible-moment-life-begins-when-s/.
5. K.E. McGrath and J. Palis, 'Hematopoiesis in the yolk sac: more than meets the eye', *Experimental Hematology* 33(9) (Sep 2005) https://www.ncbi.nlm.nih.gov/pubmed/16140150.
6. R.W. Loftin, et al., 'Late Preterm Birth', *Reviews in Obstetrics and Gynecology* 3(1) (Winter 2010): pp. 10–19. https://www.ncbi.nlm.nih.gov/pmc/articles/PMC2876317/.
7. Kirti N. Saxena, 'Anaesthesia for Fetal Surgeries', *Indian Journal of Anaesthesia* 53(5) (Oct 2009): pp. 554–9. Found at https://www.ncbi.nlm.nih.gov/pmc/articles/PMC2900087/.
8. http://www.nrlc.org/uploads/fetalpain/AnandPainReport.pdf

9. S. Sekulic, et al., 'Appearance of fetal pain could be associated with maturation of the mesodiencephalic structures', Journal of Pain Research 9 (Nov 2016): pp. 1031–8. https://www.ncbi.nlm.nih.gov/pmc/articles/PMC5115678/#!po=1.66667.
10. https://en.m.wikipedia.org/wiki/Dilation_and_evacuation.
11. https://www.gov.uk/government/uploads/system/uploads/attachment_data/file/618533/Abortion_stats_2016_commentary_with_tables.pdf.

Chapter 9: Adoption Explored
1. DfE: 'Children looked after in England year ending 31 March 2016'. https://www.gov.uk.
2. Hugh Muir, 'The Truth About Inter-Racial Adoption', The Guardian (3 Nov 2010). https://www.theguardian.com/society/2010/nov/03/inter-racial-adoption, but this was back in 2010.
3. https://www.quora.com/Do-people-generally-regret-adoption.
4. Dr Kirsty Saunders, MBChB, DCH. Adoption paediatrician.

Chapter 10: Abortion Explored
1. Taken from 'Information About Abortion Care', Royal College of Obstetricians & Gynaecologists (Feb 2012). https://www.rcog.org.uk/en/patients/patient-leaflets/abortion-care (accessed 7-8-2017).
2. M. Niinimaki, A. Pouta, et al. 'Immediate complications after medical compared with surgical termination of pregnancy', Obstetrics and Gynaecology 114(4) (Oct 2009). https://www.ncbi.nlm.nih.gov/pubmed/19888037 (accessed 07-08-2017).
3. 'The Care of Women Requesting Induced Abortion' Royal College of Gynaecologists (Nov 2011). https://www.rcog.org.uk/globalassets/documents/guidelines/abortion-guideline_web_1.pdf (accessed 10-06-2017) also http://www.patient.co.uk/health/pelvic-inflammatory-disease-leaflet (accessed 07-08-2017).
4. 'The Care of Women Requesting Induced Abortion', RCOG (Nov 2011).
5. G. Penny, 'Treatment of pain during medical abortion', Contraception 74(1) (Jul 2006): pp. 45–7.
6. Spitz, Irving, et al., 'Early Pregnancy Termination with Mifepristone and Misoprostol in the United States', The New England Journal of Medicine, 338:1241-1247 (30 Apr 1998) online (accessed 07-08-2017).
7. 'The Care of Women Requesting Induced Abortion', RCOG (Nov 2011).
8. 'The Care of Women Requesting Induced Abortion', RCOG (Nov 2011).
9. 'The Care of Women Requesting Induced Abortion', RCOG (Nov 2011).
10. S.G. Kaali, et al., 'The frequency and management of uterine perforations during first trimester abortions', American Journal of Obstetrics & Gynecology 61(2) (Aug 1989): pp. 406–8. www.ajog.org/article/0002-9378(89)90532-2/pdf (accessed 07-08-2017).
11. Reported in UK government's 'The Confidential enquiry into maternal and infant deaths' in 2008.

12. 'Abortion Care', Royal College of Obstetricians & Gynaecologists, 2012. https://www.rcog.org.uk/globalassets/documents/patients/patient-information-leaflets/pregnancy/pi-abortion-care.pdf (accessed 10-6-17).

13. P.S. Shah, J. Zao, 'Induced termination of pregnancy and low birth weight and preterm birth: a systematic review and meta-analyses, *British Journal of Obstetrics & Gynaecology* 116 (Oct 2009): pp. 1425–42. https://www.ncbi.nlm.nih.gov/pubmed/19769749 (accessed 9-8-17).

14. D. Trichopoulos, et al., 'Age at any birth and breast cancer risk', *International Journal of Cancer* 31 (15 Jun 1983): pp. 701–4. http://onlinelibrary.wiley.com/doi/10.1002/ijc.2910310604/abstract (accessed 14-6-17). Each one-year delay in FFTP increases relative breast cancer risk by 3.5%. These figures kindly interpreted and supplied by Dr Robert Dixon, medical statistician Sheffield, 3 March 2017 who added, 'One fifth or 20% is in keeping with the 95% confidence limits of 2.3% to 4.7%.'

15. 'The Care of Women Requesting Induced Abortion', RCOG (Nov 2011).

16. 'The Care of Women Requesting Induced Abortion', RCOG (Nov 2011).

17. Dr Angela Lanfranchi, Prof. Ian Gentles, Elizabeth Ring-Cassidy, *Complications: Abortion's Impact on Women* (Toronto: deVeber, 2013), p. 181.

18. D. Fergusson, L.J. Horwood and J. Boden, 'Does abortion reduce the mental health risks of unwanted or unintended pregnancy? A reappraisal of the evidence', *Australian and New Zealand Journal of Psychiatry* 47(9) (Sep 2013): pp. 819–27 https://www.ncbi.nlm.nih.gov/pubmed/23553240.

19. See also W. Pedersen, 'Abortion and depression: a population-based longitudinal study of young women', *Scandinavian Journal of Public Health* 36(4) (Jun 2008): pp. 424–8. https://www.ncbi.nlm.nih.gov/pubmed/18539697.

20. 'Induced Abortion and Mental Health'. Academy of Medical Royal Colleges (Dec 2011). https://www.aomrc.org.uk/wp-content/uploads/2016/05/Induced_Abortion_Mental_Health_1211.pdf

21. P.K. Coleman, D.C. Reardon, B.C. Calhoun, 'Reproductive History Patterns and Long-Term Mortality Rate: a Danish Population-Based Record Linkage Study', *European Journal of Public Health* 23(4) (2012):pp. 569–74. https://www.ncbi.nlm.nih.gov/pubmed/22954474.

22. C. Morgan, et al., 'Suicides After Pregnancy: Mental health may deteriorate as a direct effect of induced abortion', *British Medical Journal* 314(7084) (Mar 1997). http://www.bmj.com/content/314/7084/902.

23. M. Gissler, C. Berg, et al., 'Pregnancy associated mortality after birth, spontaneous abortion, or induced abortion in Finland, 1987–2000'. *American Journal of Obstetrics and Gynaecology* 190 (2004): pp. 422–7. https://www.ncbi.nlm.nih.gov/pubmed/14981384.

24. M. Gissler, C. Berg, et al., 'Methods for identifying pregnancy-associated deaths: Population-based data from Finland 1987–2000'. *Paediatric and Perinatal Epidemiology* 18(6) (Nov 2004): pp. 448–55. https://www.ncbi.nlm.nih.gov/pubmed/15535821.

25. 'Reproductive History Patterns and Long-Term Mortality Rate', *EJPH* (2012).

26. 'Reproductive History Patterns and Long-Term Mortality Rate', *EJPH* (2012).

27. D.C. Reardon, P.G. Ney, et al., 'Deaths associated with pregnancy outcome: A record linkage study of low income women', *Southern Medical Journal* 95(8) (Aug 2002):834–41. https://www.ncbi.nlm.nih.gov/pubmed/12190217.

28. 'Reproductive History Patterns and Long-Term Mortality Rate', *EJPH* (2012).

29. 'Reproductive History Patterns and Long-Term Mortality Rate', *EJPH* (2012).

30. https://www.hta.gov.uk/faqs/disposal-pregnancy-remains-faqs (accessed 17-7-17). Also https://www.hta.gov.uk/sites/default/files/Guidance_on_the_disposal_of_pregnancy_remains.pdf.

Chapter 11: Abortion Law in the UK and Abroad

1. Montgomery (appellant) v Lanarkshire Health Board (respondent) (2015) UKSC 11, on appeal from (2013) CSHIH 3. https://www.supremecourt.uk/decided-cases/docs/UKSC_2013_0136_Judgment.pdf.

2. GMC and BMA guidance quoted in Philippa Taylor, *Abortion: Doctors' Duties and Rights*, (London: Christian Medical Fellowship, 2016), p. 43.

3. Current Department of Health guidance on abortion provision stipulates that women must be given impartial, accurate and evidence-based information (verbal and written) delivered neutrally and covering alternatives to abortion.

4. P. Taylor, *Abortion: Doctors' Duties and Rights*, 2016.

5. An event reported to the author in the last 12 months.

6. Letter from Jeremy Hunt, the Secretary of State for Health, London, 5 September 2014 to the author.

7. Letter from General Medical Council to CEO of Christian Medical Fellowship (26 March 2008).

8. This is a typical proportion based on my own research in recent years.

9. The list of these cases is available from the author.

10. Standard for Adverse Risk Warnings: US Ninth Circuit Court ruled: 'We believe a risk must be disclosed even if it is but a potential risk rather than a conclusively determined risk. It may be that these risks had not yet been documented or accepted as a fact in the medical profession. Nonetheless, under the doctrine of informed consent, these risks should have been disclosed. Medical knowledge should not be limited to what is generally accepted by the profession.' J. Kindley, 'The Fit Between the Elements for an Informed Consent Cause of Action and the Scientific Evidence Linking Induced Abortion with Breast Cancer Risk', *Wisconsin Law Review* (1998): pp. 1595–1644. http://www.kindleylaw.com/wp-content/uploads/2009/05/1998WLR15952.pdf.

Chapter 12: Overview of the After-effects of Abortion

1. Personal discussion with an experienced schools sex and relationships specialist from Doncaster.

2. 'Abortion Care', Royal College of Obstetricians and Gynaecologists (2012). https://www.rcog.org.uk/globalassets/documents/patients/patient-information-leaflets/pregnancy/pi-abortion-care.pdf (accessed 10-6-17).

3. Dr Angela Lanfranchi, Prof. Ian Gentles, Elizabeth Ring-Cassidy, *Complications: Abortion's Impact on Women* (Toronto: deVeber, 2013), p. 170. Cited in A.J. Boeke, J.E. van Bergen et al., 'The risk of pelvic inflammatory disease associated with urogenital infection with chlamydia trachomatis; literature review', *Nederlands Tijdschrift voor Geneeskunde* 149(15) (Apr 2005): pp. 878–84. https://www.ncbi.nlm.nih.gov/pubmed/15868993.

4. D. Trichopoulos, et al., 'Age at any birth and breast cancer risk', *International Journal of Cancer* 31 (15 Jun 1983): pp. 701–4. http://onlinelibrary.wiley.com/doi/10.1002/ijc.2910310604/abstract (accessed 14-6-17). Each one-year delay in FFTP increases relative breast cancer risk by 3.5%. These figures kindly interpreted and supplied by Dr Robert Dixon, medical statistician Sheffield, 3 March 2017 who added, 'One fifth or 20% is in keeping with the 95% confidence limits of 2.3% to 4.7%.'

5. V. Beral, D. Bull, et al., 'Breast Cancer and Abortion: A collaborative reanalysis of data from 53 studies, including 83,000 women from 16 countries', *Lancet* 363(9414) (Mar 2004): pp. 1007–16. https://www.ncbi.nlm.nih.gov/pubmed/15051280.

6. These 46 studies are listed at http://www.choicescommunity.com.

7. 'The Care of Women Requesting Induced Abortion', Royal College of Gynaecologists (Nov 2011). https://www.rcog.org.uk/globalassets/documents/guidelines/abortion-guideline_web_1.

8. L. Henriet, M. Kaminski, 'Impact of induced abortions on subsequent pregnancy outcome: the 1995 French national perinatal survey', *British Journal of Obstetrics & Gynaecology* 108(10) (Oct 2001): pp. 1036–42. https://www.ncbi.nlm.nih.gov/pubmed/11702834.

9. UK Confidential Inquiry into Maternal Deaths 2008.

10. S.G. Kaali, et al., 'The frequency and management of uterine perforations during first trimester abortions', *American Journal of Obstetrics & Gynecology* 61(2) (Aug 1989): pp. 406–8. www.ajog.org/article/0002-9378(89)90532-2/pdf (accessed 07-08-2017).

11. 'The Care of Women Requesting Induced Abortion', RCOG (Nov 2011).

12. D. Yu, T.C. Li, et al., 'Factors affecting reproductive outcome of hysteroscopic adhesiolyis for Asherman's syndrome', *Fertility and Sterility* 89 (3) (Mar 2008): pp. 715–22. https://www.ncbi.nlm.nih.gov/pubmed/17681324.

13. D. Fergusson, L.J. Horwood and J. Boden, 'Does abortion reduce the mental health risks of unwanted or unintended pregnancy? A reappraisal of the evidence', *Australian and New Zealand Journal of Psychiatry* 47(9) (Sep 2013): pp. 1204–5 https://www.ncbi.nlm.nih.gov/pubmed/23553240.

14. W. Pedersen, 'Abortion and depression: a population-based longitudinal study of young women', *Scandinavian Journal of Public Health* 36(4) (Jun 2008): pp. 424–8.

https://www.ncbi.nlm.nih.gov/pubmed/18539697.

15. Cases reported to the author, or known personally to the author. Online examples and published examples are open to all to see.

16. Cases reported to the author and communications from experienced pastors and family doctors.

17. Fully covered in Dr Angela Lanfranchi, Prof. Ian Gentles, Elizabeth Ring-Cassidy, *Complications: Abortion's Impact on Women* (Toronto: deVeber, 2013), chapters 1, 17–19.

18. C. Garcia-Moreno, et al., *WHO multi-country study on women's health and domestic violence against women* (Geneva: World Health Organisation, 2005): pp. xv. http://www.who.int/gender/violence/who_multicountry_study/summary_report/summary_report_English2.pdf

19. Age-Adjusted odds ratio 95% confidence interval 1.03–18.2, p value 0.02–4.42 and not .36–9.10 respectively; M. Gissler, et al. 'Pregnancy-associated deaths in Finland 1987–1994 – definition problems and benefits of record linkage', *Acta Obstetricia et Gynecologica Scandinavica* 76 (7) (Aug 1997): pp. 651–7. https://www.ncbi.nlm.nih.gov/pubmed/9292639,

20. M.A. Hassan and S.R. Killick, 'Is previous aberrant reproductive outcome predictive of subsequently reduced fecundity?' *Human Reproduction* 20(3) (Mar 2005): pp. 657–64. Odds ratio 7.2 (p value 0.02): p. 662. Further evidence in Dr Angela Lanfranchi, Prof. Ian Gentles, Elizabeth Ring-Cassidy, *Complications: Abortion's Impact on Women* (Toronto: deVeber, 2013), p. 176.

21. 'The Care of Women Requesting Induced Abortion', RCOG (Nov 2011).

22. W. Zhou, J. Olsen, et al., 'Risk of spontaneous abortion following induced abortion is only increased with short interpregnancy interval', *Journal of Obstetrics and Gynaecology* 20(1) (Jan 2000): pp. 49–54. https://www.ncbi.nlm.nih.gov/pubmed/15512467

23. G. Xu, Y. Wu, et al., 'Risk factors for early miscarriage among Chinese: a hospital-based case-control study', *Fertility and Sterility* 101(6) (Jun 2014): pp. 1663-70. https://www.ncbi.nlm.nih.gov/pubmed/24666755. This shows a 'dose response'. Prior Induced Abortions bring raised relative odds of miscarriage as follows:
1 19% < 1.19 (1.01-1.37) >
2 61% < 1.61 (1.19-3.12) >
Over 2 156% < 2.56 (1.33-4.58) >

24. K. Mühlemann, M. Germain, M. Krohn, 'Does abortion increase the risk of intrapartum infection in the following pregnancy? *Epidemiology* 7(2) (Mar 1996): pp. 194–8. https://www.ncbi.nlm.nih.gov/pubmed/8834561.

25. C. Ooi and L. Dayan, 'Pelvic inflammatory disease: an approach for GPs in Australia', *Australian Family Physician* 32(5) (May 2003)). http://www.racgp.org.au/afpback-issues/2003/200305/20030501ooi.pdf.

26. Odds Ratio 4.79 (95% Confidence Interval 1.46–15.68); W. Zhou and J. Olsen, 'Are complications after an induced abortion associated with reproductive failures in a

subsequent pregnancy?' *Acta Obstetricia et Gynecologica Scandinavica* 82(2) (Feb 2003): 177–81. https://www.ncbi.nlm.nih.gov/pubmed/12648182.

27. L.K. Dhaliwal, K.R. Gupta and S. Gopalan, 'Induced abortion and subsequent pregnancy outcome', *Journal of Family Welfare* 49(1) (Jun 2003), pp. 50–55. https://www.popline.org/node/233271.

28. Research published June 2015 on 2 million women: https://www.sciencedaily.com/releases/2015/06/150616072331.htm.

29. P.S. Shah, J. Zao, 'Induced termination of pregnancy and low birth weight and preterm birth: a systematic review and meta-analyses, *British Journal of Obstetrics & Gynaecology* 116 (Oct 2009): pp. 1425-42. https://www.ncbi.nlm.nih.gov/pubmed/19769749 (accessed 9-8-17).

Chapter 13: Teenage Pregnancy and Abortion – Take Special Care

1. Dr Angela Lanfranchi, Prof. Ian Gentles, Elizabeth Ring-Cassidy, *Complications: Abortion's Impact on Women* (Toronto: deVeber, 2013).

2. J. Jeffes, *Unplanned Pregnancy: Talking with Teenagers* (Hove: Lean Press, 2013).

3. D.M. Fergusson, L.J. Horwood and E.M. Ridder, 'Abortion in young women and subsequent mental health', *Journal of Child Psychology and Psychiatry* 47(1) (Jan 2006), pp. 16–24. https://www.ncbi.nlm.nih.gov/pubmed/16405636.

4. G. Condon and D. Hazzard, *Fatherhood Aborted: The Profound Effects of Abortion on Men,* (Carol Stream, IL: Tyndale House, 2001). See also http://www.deveber.org/text/chapters/Chap16.pdf.

5. J. Jeffes, *Unplanned Pregnancy: Talking with Teenagers*, 2013.

6. Name known to the author MH.

7. Prof. Ian Gentles and Elizabeth Ring-Cassidy, *Women's Health after Abortion: The Medical and Psychological Evidence* (Toronto: deVeber Institute, 2002).

8. P.K. Coleman, 'Resolution of Unwanted Pregnancy During Adolescence Through Abortion Versus Childbirth: Individual and Family Predictors and Psychological Consequences,' *Journal of Youth and Adolescence* 35(6) (Dec 2006): pp.903–911.

9. B. Garfinkel, et al. 'Stress, depression and suicide: A study of adolescents in Minnesota', University of Minnesota (1986): pp. 43–55.

10. C. Morgan, M. Evans and J. Peters, 'Suicides after Pregnancy', BMJ 314(902) (Mar 1997), data extracted and plotted from Table 1, pp. 902–3.

11. D.M. Fergusson, L.J. Horwood and E.M. Ridder, 'Abortion in young women and subsequent mental health', *JCPP*, 2006.

12. N.B Campbell, K. Franco, S. Jurs, 'Abortion in Adolescence', *Adolescence*, 23(92) (Winter 1998): 813-23. https://www.ncbi.nlm.nih.gov/pubmed/3232570.

13. Personal to author January 2017.

14. R.T. Burkman, et al., 'Morbidity risk among young adolescent undergoing elective abortion', *Contraception* 30(2) (Aug 1984): pp. 99–105. https://www.ncbi.nlm.nih.gov/pubmed/6499441.

15. S. Osser and K. Perrson, 'Post Abortal Pelvic Infection Associated with Chlamydia

Trachomatis Infection and the Influence of Humoral Immunity', *American Journal of Obstetrics and Gynecology* 150(6) (Nov 1984):pp. 699–703. http://www.ajog.org/article/0002-9378(84)90670-7/fulltext.

Chapter 14: Men, Pregnancy and Abortion

1. J. Jeffes, *What Happens after an Abortion?* (Hove: Lean Press, 2014).
2. B. McMahon, 'Play fighting and straight talking: the new science on why dads matter', *The Times* (20 Jun 2015). https://www.thetimes.co.uk/article/play-fighting-and-straight-talking-the-new-science-on-why-dads-matter-ghcswlbhwlp.
3. A. Kero, A. Lalos, et al., 'The male partner involved in legal abortion', *Human Reproduction* 14(10) (Oct 1999): pp. 2669–75. http://humrep.oxfordjournals.org/content/14/10/2669.full.
4. Case reports to the author.
5. A. Lanfranchi, I. Gentles, E. Ring-Cassidy, *Complications: Abortion's Impact on Women* (Toronto: deVeber, 2013).
6. http://www.menandabortion.com/articles.html (accessed 16/4/14).
7. h http://www.menandabortion.com/articles.html (accessed 16/4/14).
8. L. Bird Franke, *The Ambivalence of Abortion* (New York: Random House, 1978), p. 63. See also, D. Reardon, *Aborted Women, Silent No More* (Good New Publishers, 1987), p. 45.
9. Dr T. Karminski Burke, 'Can Relationships Survive after Abortion?' http://afterabortion.org/1999/can-relationships-survive-after-abortion/.
10. Sharon Pearce, 'Can Relationships Survive after an Abortion?' http://www.silentvoices.org/blog/can-relationships-survive-after-an-abortion (accessed 10-7-17).

Chapter 15: Antenatal Screening and Disability in the Fetus

1. John Wyatt, *Matters of Life and Death* (Nottingham: IVP, 2nd edn, 2009), p. 84. A fetal medicine specialist writes, 'I have tried to find more accurate data about the chance of an abnormality but it is very difficult to obtain such data – is it babies born? Or is it babies diagnosed antenatally? One must ask does it include chromosome and structural anomalies – and what constitutes an anomaly? When I was discussing screening tests with women who had an increased risk of having a baby with an abnormality, because of the drugs they needed to take for medical complications, I gave them a "background" risk of 2–3% of a major abnormality, e.g. spina bifida or major cardiac defect. So, I think 1 in 25, i.e. 4% is very reasonable.' Personal communication from Dr Fiona Fairley 01-06-17, a recently retired specialist in fetal medicine, Sheffield, UK.
2. Wyatt, *Matters of Life and Death*, 2009.
3. http://www.nhs.uk/conditions/Chorionic-Villus-sampling/Pages/Introduction.aspx (accessed 14-6-17).
4. 'Non-Invasive Prenatal Testing: Ethical Issues', Nuffield Council on Bioethics (Mar 2017). http://nuffieldbioethics.org/wp-content/uploads/NIPT-ethical-issues-full-report.pdf.

5. 'Non-Invasive Prenatal Testing: Ethical Issues', Nuffield Council on Bioethics (Mar 2017).

6. National Institute for Clinical Excellence, 'Antenatal Care: Routine Care for the Healthy Pregnant Woman'. Clinical Guideline CG62, NICE (Mar 2008). http://guidance.nice.org.uk/CG62.

7. H. Statham, et al., 'Prenatal diagnosis of fetal abnormality: psychological effects on women in low risk pregnancies', *Best Practice & Research Clinical Obstetrics and Gynaecology* 14 (2000): pp. 731–47. (See J. Wyatt, *Matters of Life and Death*, ftn. 9 p. 112.)

8. R. Dodds, 'The stress of tests in pregnancy: an antenatal screening survey', National Childbirth Trust (UK), 1997. (See Prof J. Wyatt ftn. 14, p. 113.)

9. G. McGee, *The Perfect Baby*, quoted in Wyatt, *Matters of Life and Death*, 2009, p. 114.

10. V. Davies, et al. 'Psychological outcome in women undergoing termination of pregnancy for ultrasound-detected fetal anomaly in the first and 2nd trimesters: a pilot study', *Ultrasound in Obstetrics & Gynecology* 25(4) (Apr 2005): pp. 389–92. https://www.ncbi.nlm.nih.gov/pubmed/15791695.

11. Wyatt, *Matters of Life and Death*, 2009.

12. C.H. Zeanah, et al., 'Do women grieve after terminating pregnancies because of fetal anomalies? A controlled investigation', *Obstetrics & Gynecology* 82(2) (Aug 1993): pp. 270–5. https://www.ncbi.nlm.nih.gov/pubmed/8336876.

13. B.G. Skotko, et al., 'Having a son or daughter with Down syndrome: perspectives from mothers and fathers'. *American Journal of Medical Genetics Part A* 155A(10) (Oct 2011): 2,335-47. (Quoted in CMF files 63, summer 2017, https://www.christianmedicalfellowship.org.uk.) https://www.ncbi.nlm.nih.gov/pubmed/21915989.

PART 3: INFORMING CHOICE BY DIGGING DEEPER
Chapter 16: Physical After-effects of Abortion

1. M. Niinimaki, A. Pouta, et al. 'Immediate complications after medical compared with surgical termination of pregnancy', *Obstetrics and Gynaecology* 114(4) (Oct 2009). https://www.ncbi.nlm.nih.gov/pubmed/19888037 (accessed 07-08-2017). This was a 2009 study from Finland involving follow-up checks of 42,619 women.

2. 'The care of women requesting induced abortion', Royal College of Obstetricians and Gynaecologists (Nov 2011. https://www.rcog.org.uk/globalassets/documents/guidelines/abortion-guideline_web_1.pdf.

3. G. Penny, 'Treatment of pain during medical abortion', *Contraception* 74(1) (Jul 2006): pp. 45–7.

4. Spitz, Irving, et al., 'Early Pregnancy Termination with Mifepristone and Misoprostol in the United States', *The New England Journal of Medicine*, 338:1241–7 (30 Apr 1998) online (accessed 07-08-2017).

5. K.R. Meckstroth, K. Mishra, 'Analgesia/pain management in the first trimester surgical abortion', *Clinical Obstetrics and Gynecology* (Jun 2009) 52(2): pp. 160–70.

6. G. Penny, 'Treatment of pain during medical abortion', *Contraception* 74(1) (Jul 2006): pp. 45–7.

7. S. Suliman, et al., 'Comparison of pain, cortisol levels, and psychological distress in women undergoing surgical termination of pregnancy under local anaesthesia versus intravenous sedation. *BMC Psychiatry* 7(24) (Jun 2007): pp. 24–32. https://www.ncbi. nlm.nih.gov/pmc/articles/PMC1899490/.

8. A.J. Boeke, J.E. van Bergen et al., 'The risk of pelvic inflammatory disease associated with urogenital infection with chlamydia trachomatis; literature review', *Nederlands Tijdschrift voor Geneeskunde* 149(15) (Apr 2005): pp. 878–84.

9. https://www.nice.org.uk/news/article/treat-life-threatening-sepsis-within-the-hour-says-nice?utm_medium=email&utm_source=upcnewsletter&utm_campaign=sepsisdraftqsmar17 (accessed 30-3-17).

10. S. Chen, J. Li, A. van den Hoek, 'Universal screening or prophylactic treatment for Chlamydia trachomatis infection among women seeking induced abortions: which strategy is more cost-effective?' *Sexually Transmitted Diseases* 34(4) (Apr 2007): pp. 230–6. https://www.ncbi.nlm.nih.gov/pubmed/17414068.

11. S.G. Kaali, et al., 'The frequency and management of uterine perforations during first trimester abortions', *American Journal of Obstetrics & Gynecology* 61(2) (Aug 1989): pp. 406–8. www.ajog.org/article/0002-9378(89)90532-2/pdf (accessed 07-08-2017).

Chapter 17: Mortality of Women After Birth and Abortion

1. D.C. Reardon, P.K. Coleman, 'Short and long-term mortality rates associated with first pregnancy outcome: population register-based study for Denmark 1980–2004', *Medical Science Monitor* 18(9) (Sep 2012): pp. 71–6. https://www.ncbi.nlm.nih.gov/pubmed/22936199.

2. Data points from D.C. Reardon, P.K. Coleman, 'Short and long-term mortality rates associated with first pregnancy outcome: population register-based study for Denmark 1980–2004', *Medical Science Monitor* 18(9) (Sep 2012): pp. 71–6. Table 1 with 180-day data from Table 2. (This study did not control for social and financial factors, marital status and mental health before the abortion.)

3. D.C. Reardon, P.K. Coleman, 'Short and long-term mortality rates associated with first pregnancy outcome: population register-based study for Denmark 1980–2004', *Medical Science Monitor* 18(9) (Sep 2012): pp. 71–6.

4. D.C. Reardon, P.G. Ney, et al., 'Deaths associated with pregnancy outcome: A record linkage study of low income women', *Southern Medical Journal* 95(8) (Aug 2002):834–41. https://www.ncbi.nlm.nih.gov/pubmed/12190217.

5. P.K. Coleman, D.C. Reardon, B.C. Calhoun, 'Reproductive History Patterns and Long-Term Mortality Rate: a Danish Population-Based Record Linkage Study', *European Journal of Public Health* 23(4) (2012): pp. 569–74. https://www.ncbi.nlm.nih.gov/pubmed/22954474.

6. L.A. Bartlett, et al., 'Risk factors for legal induced abortion-related mortality in the

United States', *Obstetrics & Gynecology* 103(4) (Apr 2004): pp. 729-37. P. Saukko, B. Knight, Knight's Forensic Pathology 4th edn (CRC, 2015).

7. M. Gissler, C. Berg, et al., 'Injury deaths, suicides and homicides associated with pregnancy, Finland 1987–2000', *European Journal of Public Health* 15(5) (Oct 2005): pp. 459–63. https://www.ncbi.nlm.nih.gov/pubmed/16051655.

8. M. Gissler, E. Hemminki, J. Lonnqvist, 'Suicides after pregnancy in Finland, 1987–94: register linkage study', *British Medical Journal* 313 (Dec 1996): pp. 1431–34. http://www.bmj.com/content/313/7070/1431.

9. IRTAD, the International road safety group (accessed 12-7-17). How Safe Is Safe? Communicating Risk to Decision-Makers. http://www.bioss.ac.uk/topics/howsafe.html#c4.

10. M. Gissler, C. Berg, et al., 'Pregnancy associated mortality after birth, spontaneous abortion, or induced abortion in Finland, 1987–2000'. *American Journal of Obstetrics and Gynaecology* 190 (2004): pp. 422–7. https://www.ncbi.nlm.nih.gov/pubmed/14981384.

11. Table 3 of 'Reproductive History Patterns and Long-Term Mortality Rate', *EJPH* (2012).

12. 'Reproductive History Patterns and Long-Term Mortality Rate', *EJPH* (2012).

13. 'Injury deaths, suicides and homicides associated with pregnancy, Finland 1987–2000', *EJPH* 15(5) (Oct 2005).

14. 'Suicides after pregnancy in Finland, 1987–94: register linkage study', BMJ (1996).

15. D.C. Reardon, P.G. Ney, et al., 'Deaths associated with pregnancy outcome: A record linkage study of low income women', *Southern Medical Journal* 95(8) (Aug 2002): pp. 834–41. https://www.ncbi.nlm.nih.gov/pubmed/12190217.

16. M. Gissler, C Berg, et al., 'Pregnancy-associated mortality after birth, spontaneous abortion, or induced abortion in Finland, 1987–2000', *American Journal of Obstetrics & Gynecology* 190(2) (Feb 2004): pp. 422–7.

17. D.C. Reardon, P.G. Ney, et al., 'Deaths associated with pregnancy outcome: A record linkage study of low income women', *Southern Medical Journal* 95(8) (Aug 2002):834–41. https://www.ncbi.nlm.nih.gov/pubmed/12190217.

Chapter 18: Abortion and Breast Cancer – Is There a Link?

1. Office for National Statistics, Cancer Registration Statistics, England, release date May 2017. https://www.ons.gov.uk/peoplepopulationandcommunity/healthandsocialcare/conditionsanddiseases/bulletins/cancerregistrationstatisticsengland/2015#the-three-most-common-cancers-vary-by-sex-and-age-group (accessed 11-8-17).

2. https://www.breasthealthuk.com/about-breast-cancer/breast-cancer-survival-rates (accessed 14/2/17).

3. P.S. Carroll, J.S. Utshudiema, J. Rodrigues, 'The British Breast Cancer Epidemic: Trends, Patterns, Risk Factors, and Forecasting', *Journal of American Physicians and Surgeons* 22(1) (Spring 2017). Also confirmed in a letter to Patrick Carroll from Cancer

Research UK, August 8, 2017 who recalculated latest statistics to give a figure of 1 in 7.14 women, which is similar to Carroll's published paper. (Cancer Research UK round their figures up to 1 in 8 but they are reviewing this.) Adding in the in situ cancers as well gives a figure of 1 woman in 6 for lifetime risk.

4. Breast cancer risk increase due to raised age at first full-term pregnancy, 3 references:

(A) E. Negri, et al., 'Risk factors for breast cancer: pooled results from three Italian case-control studies', *American Journal of Epidemiology* 128(6) (Dec 1988): pp. 1207–15. https://www.ncbi.nlm.nih.gov/pubmed/3195562. The 'Negri' study can be considered a small meta-analysis; first full-term pregnancy after age 28 imparts 1.8 times the B.C. risk versus first full-term pregnancy under age 22.

(B) J. Wohlfahrt, M. Melbye, 'Age at Any Birth is Associated with Breast Cancer Risk', *Epidemiology* 12(1) (Jan 2001): pp. 68–73. http://journals.lww.com/epidem/Abstract/2001/01000/Age_at_Any_Birth_Is_Associated_with_Breast_Cancer.12.aspx.

(C) D. Trichopoulos, et al., 'Age at any birth and breast cancer risk', *International Journal of Cancer* 31 (15 Jun 1983): pp. 701–4. http://onlinelibrary.wiley.com/doi/10.1002/ijc.2910310604/abstract (accessed 14-6-17). Each one-year delay in FFTP increases relative breast cancer risk by 3.5%.

5. A. Lanfranchi, I. Gentles, E. Ring-Cassidy, *Complications: Abortion's Impact on Women* (Toronto: deVeber, 2013). The argument runs that all 9 strict criteria, established by Sir Austin Bradford Hill in 1964 for *causation*, are met in the Abortion–Breast Cancer research. In the infamous history of tobacco and lung cancer, it was these criteria which led to the Surgeon General in the USA placing warnings on cigarette packets, to say that they raised the risk of lung cancer.

6. V. Beral, et al. 'Collaborative Group on Hormonal Factors in Breast Cancer. Breast cancer and abortion: collaborative reanalysis of data from 53 epidemiological studies, including 83,000 women with breast cancer from 16 countries', *Lancet* 363(9414) (2004): pp. 1007–16.

7. A.R. Jiang, C.M. Gao, J.H. Ding, et al., 'Abortions and breast cancer risk in premenopausal and postmenopausal women in Jiangsu Province of China', *Asian Pacific Journal of Cancer Prevention* 13(1) (2012): pp. 33–5. Quoted in p. 115 and later in book from deVeber 2013, *Complications: Abortion's Impact on Women*, Dr Angela Lanfranchi, MD, breast surgeon, Prof Ian Gentles, Elizabeth Ring Cassidy psychologist.

8. P.S. Carroll, J.S. Utshudiema, J. Rodrigues, 'The British Breast Cancer Epidemic: Trends, Patterns, Risk Factors, and Forecasting', *Journal of American Physicians and Surgeons* 22(1) (Spring 2017).

9. Y. Huang, X. Zhang, et al., 'A meta-analysis of the association between induced abortion and breast cancer risk among Chinese females', *Cancer Causes Control* 25(2) (Feb 2014): pp. 227-36.

10. These figures kindly interpreted by Dr Robert Dixon, medical statistician Sheffield, 3 March 2017 who added, 'One fifth' is in keeping with the 95% confidence limits of 2.3% to 4.7%.'

11. D. Trichopoulos, et al., 'Age at any birth and breast cancer risk', *International Journal of Cancer* 31 (15 Jun 1983): pp. 701–4. http://onlinelibrary.wiley.com/doi/10.1002/ijc.2910310604/abstract (accessed 14-6-17). Each one-year delay in FFTP increases relative breast cancer risk by 3.5%.

12. A.B. Nilsen, U. Waldenstron, et al., 'Characteristics of women who are pregnant with their first baby at an advanced age', *Acta Obstetricia Gynecologica Scandinavica* 91(3) (Mar 2012):353–62. Comment by Prof Brent Rooney: 'This large 2012 Anne Nilsen et al. study of women in Norway looked for factors associated with "women who are pregnant with their first baby at an advanced age". The researchers subdivided their study subjects into 3 maternal age categories (25–32 years, 33–37, over age 37). If a Norwegian woman had Induced Abortion IA history, she was 70% more likely to be have a maternal age at first birth between 33 and 37 than women with no prior IAs and 90% more likely to have maternal age over 37 years than women with no prior IAs' (to the author 2017).

13. https://www.publications.parliament.uk/pa/cm200607/cmselect/cm-sctech/1045/1045we15.htm.

14. M. Melbye, J. Wohlfahrt, et al., 'Preterm delivery and risk of breast cancer', *British Journal of Cancer* 80(3/4) (May 1999): pp. 609–13. https://www.ncbi.nlm.nih.gov/pubmed/10408874.

K.E. Innes, T.E. Byers, 'First pregnancy characteristics and subsequent breast cancer risk among young women', *International Journal of Cancer* 112(2) (Nov 2004): pp. 306–11. http://onlinelibrary.wiley.com/doi/10.1002/ijc.20402/full.

15. Lecture by breast specialist Dr Iman Azmy, Chesterfield, England on 26-01-2016, figures based on the Million Women Study.

16. V. Beral, et al. 'Collaborative Group on Hormonal Factors in Breast Cancer. Breast cancer and abortion: collaborative reanalysis of data from 53 epidemiological studies, including 83,000 women with breast cancer from 16 countries', *Lancet* 363(9414) (2004): pp. 1007–16.

17. https://www.publications.parliament.uk/pa/cm200607/cmselect/cm-sctech/1045/1045we15.htm.

18. Möller, et al, 2008, 'Breast cancer and breastfeeding: collaborative reanalysis of individual data from 47 epidemiological studies in 30 countries, including 50,302 women with breast cancer and 96,973 women without the disease', *The Lancet* 360(9328) (2002): p. 187–95. https://lup.lub.lu.se/search/publication/1123899.

19. D. Wahlberg, 'Study: breast cancer not tied to abortion', *Atlanta Journal Constitution*, 26 March 2004. Quoted in A. Lanfranchi, I. Gentles, E. Ring-Cassidy, *Complications: Abortion's Impact on Women* (Toronto: deVeber, 2013).

20. The co-authors eliminated 11 studies for unscientific reasons. Thus in the end they included only 24 of the 41 studies in existence at the time of the re-analysis out of the research on induced abortion and breast cancer. To supplement these 24 studies, the researchers added a further 28 unpublished studies, not themselves having had the test of peer review nor consulted by other researchers. Readers are referred

to the full argument from which this is taken in A. Lanfranchi, I. Gentles, E. Ring-Cassi-dy, Complications: Abortion's Impact on Women (Toronto: deVeber, 2013).

21. A. Lanfranchi, I. Gentles, E. Ring-Cassidy, *Complications: Abortion's Impact on Women* (Toronto: deVeber, 2013).

22. C.C. Hsieh, J. Wuu, et al, 'Delivery of premature newborns and maternal breast-cancer risk', *The Lancet* 353(9160) (Apr 1999): p. 1239. Quoted and well explained in A. Lanfranchi, I. Gentles, E. Ring-Cassidy, *Complications: Abortion's Impact on Women* (Toronto: deVeber, 2013).

23. Black-American women who breastfeed for over 6 months cut TNBC (Triple-Negative Breast Cancer) risk by 82%. Dr H. Ma, 'Reproductive factors and the risk of triple-negative breast cancer in white women and African-American women: a pooled analysis' *Breast Cancer Research* 19(6) (Jan 2017). https://breast-cancer-research.biomedcentral.com/articles/10.1186/s13058-016-0799-9.

24. http://www.nhs.uk/Conditions/Cancer-of-the-breast-female/Pages/Causes.aspx.

25. P.S. Carroll, J.S. Utshudiema, J. Rodrigues, 'The British Breast Cancer Epidemic: Trends, Patterns, Risk Factors, and Forecasting', *Journal of American Physicians and Surgeons* 22(1) (Spring 2017). www.jpands.org/vol22no1/carroll.pdf.

26. National Cancer Registry Ireland, 2016, http://www.ncri.ie/publications/cancer-trends-and-projections/cancer-trends-29-breast-cancer (accessed 10-8-17).

27. Office of National Statistics, 2014, incidence of and mortality from malignant neoplasm of the breast 2004–2014 (accessed 10-8-17).

28. P.S. Carroll, J.S. Utshudiema, J. Rodrigues, 'The British Breast Cancer Epidemic: Trends, Patterns, Risk Factors, and Forecasting', JAPS (2017).

29. P. Carroll, *Ireland's Gain: The Demographic Impact and Consequences for the Health of Women of the Abortion Laws in Ireland and Northern Ireland*, (London: Pension and Population Research Institute, 2011).

30. 'Cancers in Northern Ireland were not regularly recorded until 1993, so the trend between 1971 and 2002 is not known with precision. Experts discuss why there are the year by year variations in cancer rates; but the way the screening programme works explains a lot of it. So, we must be careful not to read too much into any one year when comparing the British and Irish rates (both Republic and Northern Ireland).' (P. Carroll's comment to author 2017.)

31. Dr Patrick Carroll personal communication to the author 1 March 2017.

32. Carroll has most recently published on the breast cancer epidemic in spring 2017, confirming the rising numbers and abortion as part of the problem. P.S. Carroll, J.S. Utshudiema, J. Rodrigues, 'The British Breast Cancer Epidemic: Trends, Patterns, Risk Factors, and Forecasting', *Journal of American Physicians and Surgeons* 22(1) (Spring 2017).

33. M. Lambe, C. Hsieh, H. Chan, A. Ekbom, D. Trichopolous and H. Adami, 'Parity, age at first and last birth, and risk of breast cancer: a population-based study in Sweden', *Breast Cancer Research and Treatment* 38(3) (Jan 1996): pp. 305–11. https://www.

ncbi.nlm.nih.gov/pubmed/8739084.

34. *NHS breast screening: Helping you decide* (Crown copyright, 2012, for Public health England).

35. Lecture by breast specialist Dr Iman Azmy, Chesterfield, England on 26-01-2016.

36. http://breast-cancer-research.biomedcentral.com/articles/10.1186/s13058-016-0799-9.

37. M. Melbye, J. Wohlfahrt, et al., 'Induced abortion and the risk of breast cancer', *New England Journal of Medicine* 336 (1997): pp. 81–5. http://www.nejm.org/doi/full/10.1056/NEJM199701093360201#t=article.

M. Melbye, J. Wohlfahrt, et al., 'Preterm delivery and risk of breast cancer', British Journal of Cancer 80(3/4) (May 1999): pp. 609–13. https://www.ncbi.nlm.nih.gov/pubmed/10408874.

38. A. Lanfranchi, I. Gentles, E. Ring-Cassidy, *Complications: Abortion's Impact on Women* (Toronto: deVeber, 2013), p. 123.

Chapter 19: Mental and Emotional Effects of Pregnancy Loss

1. P. Taylor, *Abortion: Risks and Complications* (London: Christian Medical Fellowship, 2014).

2. 'Induced Abortion and Mental Health: A systematic review of the mental health outcomes of induced abortion, including their prevalence and associated factors' evidence-full report and consultation table with responses, Academy of Medical Royal Colleges (Dec 2011). https://www.aomrc.org.uk/wp-content/uploads/2016/05/Induced_Abortion_Mental_Health_1211.pdf.

3. D. Fergusson, L.J. Horwood and J. Boden, 'Does abortion reduce the mental health risks of unwanted or unintended pregnancy? A reappraisal of the evidence', *Australian and New Zealand Journal of Psychiatry* 47(9) (Sep 2013): pp. 1204–5 https://www.ncbi.nlm.nih.gov/pubmed/23553240.

4. See also W. Pedersen, 'Abortion and depression: a population-based longitudinal study of young women', Scandinavian Journal of Public Health 36(4) (Jun 2008): pp. 424–8. https://www.ncbi.nlm.nih.gov/pubmed/18539697.

5. D. Fergusson, L.J. Horwood and J. Boden, 'Abortion and mental health disorders: evidence from a 30-year longitudinal study', *British Journal of Psychiatry* 193(6) (Dec 2008): pp. 444–51. http://bjp.rcpsych.org/content/193/6/444.

6. D. Fergusson, L.J. Horwood and J. Boden, 'Does abortion reduce the mental health risks of unwanted or unintended pregnancy? A reappraisal of the evidence', *Australian and New Zealand Journal of Psychiatry* 47(9) (Sep 2013): pp. 1204–5 https://www.ncbi.nlm.nih.gov/pubmed/23553240.

7. 'Induced Abortion and Mental Health', AoMRC (Dec 2011).

8. B. Major, M. Applebaum, L. Beckman, et al., 'Report of the APA Task Force on Mental Health and Abortion', American Psychological Association (2008). http://www.apa.org/pi/women/programs/abortion/mental-health.pdf

9. C. Morgan, M. Evans and J. Peters, 'Suicides after Pregnancy: Mental health may

deteriorate as a direct effect of induced abortion', BMJ 314(902) (Mar 1997), data extracted and plotted from Table 1, pp. 902–3.

10. Table from the BMJ above and analysed by medical statistician Dr R. Dixon, 07-07-17.

11. A. Lanfranchi, I. Gentles, E. Ring-Cassidy, *Complications: Abortion's Impact on Women* (Toronto: deVeber, 2013).

Chapter 20: Infertility After Abortion

1. http://www.who.int/reproductivehealth/topics/infertility/definitions/en/.

2. http://www.nhs.uk/conditions/Infertility/Pages/Introduction.aspx (accessed 24-5-17).

3. M.A. Hassan and S.R. Killick, 'Is previous aberrant reproductive outcome predictive of subsequently reduced fecundity?' *Human Reproduction* 20(3) (Mar 2005): pp. 657–64. Odds ratio 7.2 (p value 0.02): p. 662. Further evidence in Dr Angela Lanfranchi, Prof. Ian Gentles, Elizabeth Ring-Cassidy, Complications: Abortion's Impact on Women (Toronto: deVeber, 2013), p. 176.

4. Y. Che, W. Zhou, E. Gao, J. Olsen, 'Induced abortion and prematurity in a subset pregnancy: a study from Shanghai', *Journal of Obstetrics and Gynaecology* 21(3) (Jul 2001): pp. 270–3. http://www.tandfonline.com/doi/abs/10.1080/01443610120046396.

5. The relative risk was 2.1, 95% confidence interval 1.1–4.0 after one previous abortion, and relative risk 2.3, 95% confidence interval 1.0–5 point 2:03 previous abortions. A. Tzonou, C.C. Hsieh, D. Trichopoulos, et al., 'Induced abortions, miscarriages, and tobacco smoking as risk factors for secondary infertility', *Journal of Epidemiology and Community Health* 47(1) (Feb 1993): pp. 36–9.

6. Hassan and Killick, 'Is previous aberrant reproductive outcome predictive of subsequently reduced fecundity?' *Human Reproduction* 2005. Also Lanfranchi, Gentles, Ring-Cassidy, *Complications: Abortion's Impact on Women*, deVeber 2013.

7. 'The care of women requesting induced abortion', Royal College of Obstetricians and Gynaecologists (Nov 2011. https://www.rcog.org.uk/globalassets/documents/guidelines/abortion-guideline_web_1.pdf.

8. W. Zhou, J. Olsen, et al., 'Risk of spontaneous abortion following induced abortion is only increased with short interpregnancy interval', *Journal of Obstetrics and Gynaecology* 20(1) (Jan 2000): pp. 49–54. https://www.ncbi.nlm.nih.gov/pubmed/15512467.

9. K. Mühlemann, M. Germain, M. Krohn, 'Does abortion increase the risk of intrapartum infection in the following pregnancy? *Epidemiology* 7(2) (Mar 1996): pp. 194–8. https://www.ncbi.nlm.nih.gov/pubmed/8834561.

10. L. Dyan, 'Pelvic inflammatory disease', *Australian Family Physician* 35(11) (2006): p. 861. Quoted in *Complications: Abortion's Impact on Women*, deVeber, 2013, p. 178.

11. *Complications: Abortion's Impact on Women*, deVeber, 2013.

12. L. Dyan, 'Pelvic inflammatory disease', *Australian Family Physician* 35(11) (2006): p. 861. Quoted in *Complications: Abortion's Impact on Women*, deVeber, 2013, p. 178.

13. Odds Ratio 4.79 (95% Confidence Interval 1.46–15.68); W. Zhou and J. Olsen, 'Are complications after an induced abortion associated with reproductive failures in a subsequent pregnancy?' *Acta Obstetricia et Gynecologica Scandinavica* 82(2) (Feb 2003): 177–81. https://www.ncbi.nlm.nih.gov/pubmed/12648182.

14. W. Zhou and J. Olsen, 'Are complications after an induced abortion associated with reproductive failures in a subsequent pregnancy?' *AOGS* 2003.

15. L.K. Dhaliwal, K.R. Gupta and S. Gopalan, 'Induced abortion and subsequent pregnancy outcome', *Journal of Family Welfare* 49(1) (Jun 2003), pp. 50–5. https://www.popline.org/node/233271.

16. *Complications: Abortion's Impact on Women*, deVeber, 2013.

17. *Complications: Abortion's Impact on Women*, deVeber, 2013, p. 167.

18. *Complications: Abortion's Impact on Women*, deVeber, 2013, p. 181.

Chapter 21: Premature Birth After Abortion

1. K.L. Costeloe, E.M. Hennessy, et al., 'Short-term outcomes after extreme preterm birth in England: comparison of two birth cohorts in 1995 and 2006 (the EPICure studies) *British Medical Journal* 345(e7976) (Dec 2012). http://www.bmj.com/content/345/bmj.e7976.

2. T. Moore, E.M. Hennessy, et al., 'Neurological and developmental outcome in extremely preterm children born in England in 1995 and 2006 (the EPICure studies) *British Medical Journal* 345(e7961) (Dec 2012). http://www.bmj.com/content/345/bmj.e7961.

3. P.S. Shah, J. Zao, 'Induced termination of pregnancy and low birth weight and preterm birth: a systematic review and meta-analyses, *British Journal of Obstetrics & Gynaecology* 116 (Oct 2009): pp. 1425–42. https://www.ncbi.nlm.nih.gov/pubmed/19769749 (accessed 9-8-17).

4. G. Saccone, L. Perriera, V. Berghella, 'Prior uterine evacuation of pregnancy as independent risk factor for preterm birth: a systematic review and meta-analysis', *American Journal Obstetrics & Gynecology* 214(5) (May 2016): pp. 572–91. http://www.ajog.org/article/S0002-9378(15)02596-X/abstract.

5. E. Lieberman, K.J. Ryan, R.R. Monson, S.C. Schoenbaum, 'Risk Factors Accounting for Racial Differences in the rate of premature birth', *New England Journal of Medicine* 317(12) (Sep 1987):743–8. http://www.nejm.org/doi/pdf/10.1056/NEJM198709173171206.

6. H.M. Swingle, T.T. Colaizy, M.B. Zimmerman, F.H. Morriss, 'Abortion and the risk of subsequent preterm birth', *Journal of Reproductive Medicine* 54(2) (Feb 2009): pp. 95–108. https://www.ncbi.nlm.nih.gov/pubmed/19301572.

7. C. Moreau, M. Kaminski, P.Y. Ancel, et al., 'Previous induced abortion and the risk of very preterm delivery: results of the EPIPAGE study', *British Journal of Obstetrics*

& *Gynaecology* 112(4) (Apr 2005): pp. 430–7. https://www.ncbi.nlm.nih.gov/pubmed/15777440.

8. K. Mühlemann, M. Germain, M. Krohn, 'Does abortion increase the risk of intrapartum infection in the following pregnancy? *Epidemiology* 7(2) (Mar 1996): pp. 194–8. https://www.ncbi.nlm.nih.gov/pubmed/8834561.

9. P.Y. Ancel, et al., 'History of induced abortion as a risk factor for preterm birth in European countries: results of the EUROPOP survey', *Human Reproduction* 19(3) (Mar 2004): pp. 734–40. https://www.ncbi.nlm.nih.gov/pubmed/14998979.

10. Ancel, et al., 'History of induced abortion as a risk factor for preterm birth in European countries' *Human Reproduction*, 2004.

11. B.C. Calhoun, E. Shadigian, B. Rooney, 'Cost consequences of induced abortion as an attributable risk for preterm birth and impact on informed consent', *Journal of Reproductive Medicine* 52(10) (Oct 2007): pp. 929–37. https://www.ncbi.nlm.nih.gov/pubmed/17977168.

Appendix 1: ABC of Spiritual Beliefs on Pregnancy and Abortion

1. H.G. Koenig, D.E. King, V. Benner Carson, *Handbook of Religion and Health* (New York: Oxford University Press, 2nd edn).

2. Jonathan Haidt examines these instinctive moral foundations in all cultures in his 2013 book *The Righteous Mind: Why Good People are Divided by Politics and Religion* (Pantheon 2012).

3. http://www.prolifehumanists.org/.

4. https://www.reddit.com/r/DebateAnAtheist/comments/2tuqix/when_does_human_life_begin/ (accessed 10-8-17).

5. https://www.reddit.com/r/DebateAnAtheist/comments/2tuqix/when_does_human_life_begin/ (accessed 10-8-17).

6. http://www.businessdictionary.com/definition/utilitarianism.html (accessed 14-6-17).

7. Taken from D. Gill, *World Religions: The essential reference guide to the world's major faiths*, (London: HarperCollins, 2003).

8. A. Lanfranchi, I. Gentles, E. Ring-Cassidy, *Complications: Abortion's Impact on Women* (Toronto: deVeber, 2013).

9. http://www.bbc.co.uk/religion/religions/buddhism/buddhistethics/abortion.shtml (accessed 17-5-17).

10. http://www.bbc.co.uk/religion/religions/buddhism/buddhistethics/abortion.shtml (accessed 17-5-17).

11. Scripture taken from the Holy Bible, New International Version (Anglicised edition) copyright ©1979, 1984, 2011 by Biblica. Used by permission of Hodder & Stoughton, an Hachette UK company. All rights reserved.

12. The earliest church fathers made abortion forbidden. It was Augustine in later times who lapsed into philosophical speculation about when the soul was present in the unborn person.

While the biblical position on the sanctity of life from conception is clear, twentieth-century Christians have been misled by inaccurate translations of the Bible verses: Exodus 21:22–25 which made Christians think God attached less value to a miscarriage, which caused a fight, than to a full-term baby born dead as the result of the fight. The correct translation of the original Hebrew is captured by the New International Version (NIV Study Bible, 2011) saying, 'If people are fighting and hit the pregnant woman and she gives birth prematurely but there is no serious injury, the offender must be fined whatever the woman's husband demands and the court allows. But if there is serious injury, you are to take life for life, tooth for tooth, hand for hand, foot for foot, burn for burn, wound for wound, bruise for bruise.' So, a dead baby in miscarriage meant the death penalty as life for life, even if the miscarriage caused by the fight was very young.

The New American Standard Bible, based on the Septuagint version rather than original Hebrew, says, 'And *if* men struggle with each other and strike a woman with child so that she has a miscarriage, yet there is no *further* injury, he shall surely be fined as the woman's husband may demand of him'. This repeat of much older mistranslations shows where the error came into the thinking of some Christians. (Scripture taken from the NEW AMERICAN STANDARD BIBLE®, Copyright © 1960,1962,1963,1968,1971,1972,1973,1975,1977 by The Lockman Foundation.) I am indebted to Revd Dr Ben Cooper for researching this for me.

13. http://www.bbc.co.uk/religion/religions/hinduism/hinduethics/abortion_1.shtml (accessed 10-8-17).
14. http://www.bbc.co.uk/religion/religions/islam/islamethics/abortion_1.shtml (accessed 10-8-17).
15. Dr Katrina Riddell, *Islam and the Secularisation of Population Policies: Muslim States and Sustainability* (London: Ashgate, 2009).
16. Shaleena's full story can be found in Angela Lanfranchi, Ian Gentles, Elizabeth Ring-Cassidy, *Complications: Abortion's Impact on Women* (Toronto: deVeber, 2013), p. 320.
17. http://www.bbc.co.uk/schools/gcsebitesize/rs/death/sikhbeliefrev2.shtml (accessed 10-8-17).
18. http://www.nhs-chaplaincy-spiritualcare.org.uk/MultiFaith/multifaithresourcefor-healthcarechaplains.pdf (accessed 11-11-15).
19. Scripture taken from the Holy Bible, New International Version (Anglicised edition) copyright ©1979, 1984, 2011 by Biblica. Used by permission of Hodder & Stoughton, an Hachette UK company. All rights reserved.
20. Scripture taken from the Holy Bible, New International Version (Anglicised edition) copyright ©1979, 1984, 2011 by Biblica. Used by permission of Hodder & Stoughton, an Hachette UK company. All rights reserved.

Further Resources and Reading

It is surprisingly difficult to find balanced sources of information on abortion decision-making. I feel the countless people of the general public, who really need quality information, are deafened by the noise from the pro- and anti-abortion camps. Many of the websites mentioned in this book and the endnotes have other good information.

The film called *HUSH*, is easy to watch and has valuable facts that the public should know, and I have checked many of these with experts.

HUSH – a liberating conversation about abortion and women's health. Director Punam Kumar Gill. Mighty Motion Pictures/Mighty Distributors Inc. 2016.

For professionals and patients the booklet called, *Abortion – Doctors Duties and Rights* (London: Christian Medical Fellowship, 2016) by Philippa Taylor will inform professionals and patients about many practical aspects of where they stand in the UK law.